DRUG ABUSE

A DAILY OCCURRENCE.

GANIHU ONYEBUASHI

CONTENTS

INTRODUCTION

Drug abuse is a very common thing in the United States and around the world. It is defined as the use of psychoactive drugs that alters one's sense of well-being and mood. A drug may be legal or illegal, but the effects are always the same. There are many different types of drugs people can abuse such as alcohol, cocaine, marijuana, and many more. The effects of drug abuse can be both physical and mental. So far about 27 million people all over the world abuse drugs. However, most of these people are abused prescription drugs rather than illegal ones. According to Center for Disease Control's National Vital Statistics Report in 2009 one out of every ten deaths was caused by drug overdose. This proves the extent to which drug abuse has reached and how dangerous it really is.

The main reason people abuse drugs is because they feel as if it will make them happier and more relaxed. They do not realize the possible harm they are doing to their bodies. They think a substance such as crack or heroin will help them cope with their problems but in real life, it only makes them worse. Drugs can also be used to escape reality for a short time. If one is feeling depressed or other emotions they can abuse drugs and use the drug to hide these feelings for a period of time. This is how people deal with their emotions rather than facing them head on. They begin to use the substance to cope with their problems and then they want to take more and more of that substance just to have a better high. But since they are on a high they do not realize the harmful effects this drug abuse has on their bodies.

Marijuana, cocaine, and heroin are known as the most commonly abused drugs in the United States. The reason these is because of how they make people feel. They are what some may call "feel good" drugs. However, there are other drugs that user's abuse that actually can cause some to have a better high which can lead to addiction. For example, the nicotine and alcohol were added into cigarettes and liquor for many people. These users of cigarettes and liquor do not realize this is part of their addiction. The more they use drugs the more addicted they become to them.

The drug abuse epidemic is not a problem that can just be solved with a solution. It cannot be solved with rapid fixes or by doing something different with the addiction. It must be treated the same as any other disorder or disease and must be treated properly in order for its patients to survive and keep their lives together in order for them to keep living healthy and happy lives.

Drug abuse is a growing epidemic that needs to be stopped now. It is becoming hard to find the root of the problem because prescription drug abuse is becoming more common and it is hard to tell when a person's addiction has reached a point where they need help from rehab, psychotherapy, or medical treatment. Without these things in place, people will continue to abuse drugs and the addiction will grow worse.

In this book, it will focus on an addiction's rise and fall, its effects, and how it is dealt with in society. The book will also focus on the different types of drugs one can abuse and why they feel the need to do this. It will also talk about the history of drug abuse, how it became so popular in society, and why people continue to abuse drugs.

The book will discuss the different types of drugs we use, which are alcohol, tobacco, marijuana, cocaine, heroin, and many others. The way these drugs affect the mind and body tissues and what changes occur to them when they abuse them. This book will also focus on how growing up with addiction in a family can affect one's life and if growing up in an alternative family can help with solving drug abuse issues.

It will also discuss the different drug abuse programs one can go through to receive help and try to kick the addiction. It will also cover the different medications people can get in order to help with their addiction and focus on how these drugs work. It will cover this information so that individuals might know what their options are if they need help with their addiction.

1

WHAT IS DRUG ABUSE?

Drug abuse is the use of an illegal or controlled substance in a manner that endangers the user or others. For example, people who take drugs to feel better, get another high, and withdraw are abusing drugs. Drug abuse can also refer to the use of legal medications that have been prescribed for a legitimate medical condition, but used without a prescription in a manner that is harmful.

People who are abusing prescription medications might be taking a higher dose than they are supposed to or having side effects that could indicate the development of an addiction problem.

There are a variety of drugs that can be abused including cocaine, methamphetamines, PCP (phencyclidine), heroin, and marijuana. Some drugs such as club drugs, which are used in social settings, are also considered to be abused.

Drug abuse can result in serious consequences for the user and for those around them. For example, it can cause withdrawal symptoms, which are unpleasant and require professional treatment to avoid potentially life-threatening issues. Drug abuse can also lead to the development of an addiction problem, which is a chronic disease that requires long-term support.

Drug abuse is often viewed as a social issue rather than a medical issue, but it can have serious long-term effects on people who make poor decisions regarding their substance use in the present. The most important goal in treating drug abuse is to get people to seek professional treatment for their addiction problem.

Drug abuse can occur at any time, but it is more likely to occur in young adults. For example, drug use can begin with experimentation during high school or college and then continue into adulthood. It can also begin during childhood and teenage years. However, it is not unusual for drugs to be present in someone's life for many years before they are actually abusing them.

Some people make poor decisions regarding drug use because they feel a need for peer approval. Drug abuse can also occur because of other social factors such as stress from school and/or family problems. Drugs may also be a form of self-medication to deal with physical or emotional pain.

Drugs are often used at parties and clubs, and this kind of environment can encourage people to try drugs for the first time. Young adults might also learn that drugs have a temporary high and then the effects go away, so they believe that drug abuse will never be a problem long-term. Drugs might also be present because of unsafe neighborhoods and schools. For example, people can use drugs to deal with the stress that comes from living in a neighborhood that doesn't have adequate resources or adequate police protection. This leads to an environment where drug abuse can occur, and it can lead to other issues such as violent crimes, thefts, and other criminal activity.

The illegal use of drugs is actually an issue of public safety. In addition to the potential danger to the user, drug abuse can lead to money being used in ways that are not productive and illegal. For example, people might steal money from their families or break into a store to steal items such as alcohol or cigarettes. Illicit drugs can also be dangerous and can lead someone to develop an addiction problem.

In addition to how drug abuse happens, it can be difficult to treat because of the unique nature of each individual.

A person who is abusing drugs might not recognize that they have a problem. For example, they might believe that the drugs are helping them to cope with stress and other issues. They might also believe that they are in control and are able to stop using them at any time.

Drug abusers can also have other mental health issues as well as physical health problems. For example, they might have anxiety or depression that is being treated with drugs such as antidepressants. In addition, physical health problems can also be treated with prescription medications and these issues can contribute to drug abuse.

Drug abuse can also be a constant cycle of abuse and sobriety, which might involve periods of abstinence followed by the use of drugs again. For example, a person might use for a few weeks and then stop for a while. They might then go a few weeks without drugs before starting again.

Drug abuse can affect a person's mental and physical health. For example, when someone is abusing drugs long-term, they might become physically dependent on the substances. This makes it difficult to stop using the substance. If someone is physically dependent on drugs, they must continue to use them to feel normal or face serious withdrawal symptoms.

Withdrawal symptoms can be difficult to be managed and cause people to feel like they need the drug just to feel normal again. For example, heroin withdrawal symptoms include vomiting, diarrhea, muscle pain, and a runny nose. It is considered a medical emergency if someone who has been abusing a drug is experiencing withdrawal symptoms.

Drug abuse can also have an impact on the development of an addiction problem. People who are addicted to drugs might experience tolerance and cravings for their substances. Tolerance is when a person feels like they need to take higher doses of the drug to feel its effects, and cravings occur when they think about using drugs or experience a desire to use the drug.

CHEMICAL AND PHYSICAL PROPERTIES OF A DRUG

The chemical and physical properties of a drug are the factors that determine how a drug will be absorbed by the body. These properties vary from drug to drug based on both the type of chemical compound and on how it is broken down in the body.

Drugs can be classified as depressants, stimulants, narcotics or hallucinogens. Depressants reduce brain activity and function; stimulants increase brain activity and function; narcotics are used to relieve pain; and hallucinogens cause the user to experience hallucinations. Another way of classifying drugs is by their chemical makeup, for example: alkaloids, peptides, proteins, or esters. It is useful in classifying drug groups that have similar characteristics because they have a similar chemical makeup.

Drugs that are systemic pass through the body. Drugs given intravenously (IV) are very effective at reaching all parts of the body, especially the brain, but also have a high risk of causing adverse effects or overdose (like excessive sleepiness and unconsciousness). The speed at which a drug hits its target depends on its route of administration. Drugs that are given orally reach their target within an hour or two. Drugs that are inhaled reach their target within minutes, and drugs that are applied to a certain area of skin may take as long as a few days to reach their target.

An important aspect of pharmacology is the description of the biological properties of drugs, which includes how they act at sites of action in the body (and in some cases, certain tissues or organs) and how these actions change over time. These properties mainly depend on the chemical composition of the drug and its physical state (for example, crystal form or solubility). The crystal form is important in many cases, especially for drugs that have polymorphic forms.

The principal chemical classification of drugs is based on the drug's chemical composition. For example, a drug can be classified as an alkaloid, a peptide or similar. These are useful in describing similar characteristics because all of these compounds share a similar chemical composition regardless of their origin (natural or synthetic) or route of administration.

The chemical classification of drugs is very broad, and it is further sub-classified. The main sub-classifications are steroids, amines, amides, ureas and nitrites. The classification of drugs into these groups is based on the drug's chemical composition. For example, a steroid can be defined as any compound that contains a cyclopentanophenanthrene ring structure. This definition includes hundreds of compounds; however, its purpose is to group all steroids together because they have similar physical and chemical properties.

The physical properties of a drug are the properties that a user can observe. These properties include the appearance of the drug, its smell, taste, and texture. This is important in defining how a drug must be handled and prepared for use. For example, if a drug has an unpleasant taste or odor then it may be taken with food or vinegar to hide these qualities. Drugs have no color or smell in their pure state but they do possess color and smell when they are added to certain chemicals. For example, if a drug is added to saline it will appear pale yellow, and if it is added to hydrogen peroxide it will appear colorless or as a dark pink color.

The physical properties of a drug are also important in defining how a drug must be administered. For example, a drug that is used intravenously must be given through a needle and syringe as it decomposes and becomes dangerous when exposed to air. The physical properties of a drug are of great importance in understanding how to treat the effects (or abuse) caused by it.

The way in which drugs are prepared affects the way they work. For example, drugs taken orally have quick-acting effects compared to those taken intravenously, or by inhalation. Drugs such as cocaine, heroin, and methamphetamine require additional processing to be absorbed into the blood. This further influences their effects; for example, when intravenously injected, cocaine will give more rapid onset of action compared to oral administration.

The capacity for a drug to cross membranes is important in understanding how it can be abused or abused safely. For example: a drug that can readily cross membranes will be absorbed quickly by the brain leading to an immediate effect. On the other hand, a drug that does not readily cross membranes will take longer for it to be absorbed into the body and thus have a slower onset of action.

The therapeutic index (or safety index) is the ratio of a drug's lethal dose to its effective dose. This is important in understanding the differences in effects caused by drugs. A drug with a high toxicity is defined as having a low therapeutic index. On the other hand, a drug that has little or no side effects is defined as having a high toxicity. A high therapeutic index means that it will have fewer side effects than a drug with an extremely low therapeutic index. For example, if an oral dose of cocaine is taken by mouth, one would say that it has low toxicity when compared to intravenous administration because the amount of cocaine required to have the same effect (i.e. produce a high) is much more when taken by mouth.

Several factors affect the pharmacokinetics of a drug. For example, the route of administration describes how a drug is taken into the body, and some routes are better for certain drugs (e.g. intravenous versus oral). The way in which a drug is taken can affect its bioavailability and thus its effects on the user or patient; sometimes adulterants are added to drugs to increase profits for producers (e.g. cocaine being sold as pure heroin).

The source of a drug can be an important factor in its chemical properties and its effects. For example, caffeine in coffee affects people differently from the same amount consumed in tea. The difference between these two sources of caffeine is due to the processing of the drug; for example, less caffeine is lost when processing coffee than when processing tea. This leads to different concentrations of caffeine in the plant material and thus different amounts ingested by users.

The detergent used in processing a drug can also affect its properties and its effects. For example, drugs that have a lipid solubility can become insoluble when processed with solvents, such as water, since they dissolve fats as well. This is important in understanding how drugs are used, as well as their abuse potential.

Some drugs require additional processing before they can be used by patients or abusers of them. This may be done for several reasons: to create a more concentrated form of the drug (e.g. cocaine in its powder form), to alter the chemical properties of the drug or to increase its bioavailability (e.g.

ephedrine, an epinephrine analog used among athletes, is often sold as a purer form of epinephrine than commercially available preparations).

Some drugs can become less potent if they are changed in any way, such as by being manufactured at a lower temperature or by performing a certain chemical reaction on them. However, other drugs are more potent after they have been processed in this way (e.g. cocaine is less potent when sold as the hydrochloride salt than when sold as coca leaves).

Some drugs become more toxic if they are mixed with certain chemicals, such as solvents or other drugs. For example, the purity of some illicit drugs can be increased by dissolving them in a solvent and then removing this solvent from the solution by evaporation (e.g. "freebasing" cocaine or heroin).

Some drugs are inhaled as part of a drug-taking session, and their chemical effects (and toxicity) are then determined by the form in which they are breathed in (e.g. "smoking" opium). Other abused drugs, including some that have never been smoked or snorted (e.g. "vaping") are taken by injection after being diluted with a solvent so that they can be absorbed more quickly into the bloodstream (e.g. intravenous drug users).

Some drugs, like heroin and cocaine, have many different forms (e.g. powder, crystaline form, and the liquid solution) that are used for purposes of abuse. Other drugs are not typically abused at all in their pure form but can be if they are processed in some way (e.g. methamphetamine).

Dependence is a result of prolonged substance use as well as other psychological and social conditions that occur when substance use is repeated over time. The effects of a drug on the brain include reduced attention, lowered inhibitions, a decrease in the ability to make decisions (e.g. impulsivity), and physical dependences (e.g. constipation or addiction).

The effects of dependency can be compared to those from withdrawal and chronic use of substances such as alcohol or drugs such as benzodiazepines because both increase anxiety and depression. Chronic use of opiates, benzodiazepines or alcohol may be also associated with mood changes. These mood changes may be very serious and lead to addiction.

PSYCHOLOGICAL AND SOCIAL EFFECTS OF DRUG ABUSE

Drug abuse is a devastating condition that can lead to serious mental health issues and other consequences. Drug abuse is a type of addiction, and since addiction is largely psychological in nature, the effects on your mind will be no less profound than those on your body. Regular users of drugs such as cocaine or heroin often turn to these substances because they have the ability to make them feel good about themselves or happy for a short time. The good feelings are endorphins which are designed to reward you for certain behaviors. These drugs are highly addictive and have a strong effect on the brain.

The psychological effects of drug use are predominantly negative as they lead to an addiction that often cripples the ability to function in society. The social consequences of abuse impact family, friends, and coworkers as well because the addicted person may neglect their responsibilities and focus around gaining access to drugs instead. As drug use becomes more frequent, users begin to withdraw from their normal daily lives to the point of neglecting even basic necessities like putting gas in the car and taking out the trash.

Drug abuse affects the brain, especially the dopamine pathway, which is involved in higher functions such as reward and motivation, pleasure and feelings of pleasure. This pathway is also influenced by drugs like cannabis and cocaine. Cocaine has been shown to damage the dopamine pathway, which can create various effects on body functions. For instance, cocaine can make the brain more excitable and able to experience euphoria. Cocaine is also an appetite suppressant, which means users are less likely to eat as they experience more intense highs and can also be more impulsive. Extreme cases of cocaine addiction may present with paranoia, delusions, hallucinations, and even suicidal thoughts.

When dopamine function is altered by drugs such as cocaine and methamphetamine, the brain gets rewired so that drug abuse becomes a central and necessary part of life. Drug use becomes all-consuming for those with an addiction. It takes over family life, relationships with friends, school or work responsibilities...any activity that is not drug-related becomes completely unimportant to the addict.

In addition to changing the physical brain structure, the drug user's personality and morals begin to change. The most usual effects of drug abuse include "out-of-character" behavior, memory loss, anxiety, depression, hyperactivity, and an increased risk for violence. These physical and psychological changes can have a major impact on family life as well. A person with an addiction may not want to care for their family, such as hygiene or putting on pants. Drug abusers may also be prone to violence and abusive behavior.

You can also have the physical health consequences of drug abuse. Depending on the individual, these problems can include diseases such as hepatitis or HIV and liver failure. This is because drugs cause users to neglect their personal health care, which may lead to serious infections that cannot be treated effectively.

Both mental and physical health may be affected by drug addiction, but they are not necessarily connected. To further complicate things, people vary in how sensitive they are to regard psychological effects of drugs as well as develop tolerance for the effects at different rates. This means that a person may experience highly psychological effects of drugs yet be physically well off while their friend, who is also psychologically sensitive, can have mental and physical health problems.

Other than the negative effects on the body's own processes, drug abuse has a tendency to cause social problems. Drug users often make poor decisions and do not think about anything beyond their next fix.

Better choices can lead to more stable lives that are consistent with family obligations and responsibilities.

Having a drug addiction can cause numerous social problems in a person's life. Some of the most common effects are on relationships with friends and family, which can be severely damaged by such an addiction. Drug addicts often neglect their family and friends in favor of seeking out drugs. Not only that but they can also be violent towards them as well.

In extreme cases, drug abuse may lead to homelessness as users simply cannot keep a job or maintain stable housing.

This can be due to drug-caused brain damage or the inability to function on a daily basis. Home drug use may also lead to criminal behavior such as theft, robbery, and other misdeeds because of the impulsive nature of drug addiction.

A person with drug addiction will be unable to participate in any activities that involve important personal relationships, such as sports, if they are too reliant on drugs to feel normal.

The most crucial thing to remember about social effects of drug abuse is that the person who abuses drugs will find it extremely difficult to sustain a fully functional life while they are addicted. This can interfere with their ability to maintain employment or to take care of themselves properly, which can lead to health problems.

Addiction to drugs is a problem that is constantly growing over in the United States. In fact, there were about 20 million people addicted to drugs in the 1980s and it is estimated that number has grown by 4 million. Because of all of the negative effects drug use can have on our society, it is important for us to recognize this epidemic as we can help reduce the amount of people who are suffering from it and maybe one day we will be able to eliminate this devastating disease entirely.

FEW COMMONLY ABUSED DRUGS

There are many types of drugs abused by Americans. Some are legal in the United States, but their abuse is still illegal. Others are considered to be illegal at all times.

Alcohol (legal): The most common legal drug in the United States, alcohol is found in beverages ranging from beer and wine to distill spirits like whiskey and vodka. People drink it for a number of reasons: to have fun with friends; to relieve stress; or just because it's available and they have the money for it. Alcohol is also used to deal with problems like anxiety, depression, and stomach upset. Alcoholism is a disease that can cause psychological and physical damage if left untreated.

Nicotine (illegal): Nicotine is an alkaloid extracted from tobacco leaves. Tobacco use is on the rise in the United States because of the popularity of cigarettes, cigars, chewing tobacco, snuff, and pipes. The nicotine in these products comes from the tobacco plant itself or from chemical additives which are added to some tobacco products. Nicotine is addictive, meaning that it causes physical dependence. The nicotine in tobacco products may cause cancer and heart disease.

Like alcohol and nicotine, illegal drugs have a chemical composition that makes them mind-altering. By changing the manner they interact with the brain and nervous system, they can produce sensations of euphoria or heightened alertness or both. If used in excess, they can impair mental function, leading to memory loss and behavioral problems. Some illegal drugs are so powerful that even small doses can cause death.

Cocaine (illegal): Cocaine is a crystalline powder derived from the leaves of the coca plant. It is used in a variety of drugs, including crack and powder cocaine. A person may use cocaine recreationally or to achieve euphoria or to lift moods with its capacity to produce feelings of self-confidence and well-being. Cocaine also acts like an appetite suppressant, making people feel full after eating very little food. In small doses, it may induce euphoria. Overdoses, however, cause cardiac arrest and severe respiratory distress.

Caffeine (illegal): Caffeine is found in beverages such as coffee, tea, soft drinks, and energy drinks. The drug acts as a stimulant by acting on sympathetic nervous system activity and the central nervous system (the part of the brain which controls voluntary movement). If taken in high amounts, caffeine creates a jittery sensation because it affects an area of the brain that regulates muscle movement.

Cannabis (legal): The primary active chemical in cannabis is THC, which produces feelings of euphoria, relaxation, and increased sensitivity to touch. Some users report intense altered states of consciousness that lead them to forget their problems and their surroundings. Cannabis is the dried leaves and flowering tops of the hashish plant. Marijuana is dried leaves and flowering tops of cannabis plants that have been specially cultivated to increase THC content. Hashish is the resin extracted from the cannabis plant. The chemicals in cannabis vary according to the resin, the plant, and the growing conditions. Today marijuana is legal in twenty-three states for medical purposes. Synthetic cannabinoids that act on the endocannabinoid system are also legal in many states.

Cough (illegal): Cough is most commonly used by athletes as a form of performance enhancing drug to increase their endurance and enhance their oxygen uptake. It has been used by athletes in many sports including swimming, track and field, cycling, football, professional wrestling and mixed martial arts as well as bodybuilding. It is a stimulant drug and is extremely addictive, with many serious side effects.

Methamphetamine (illegal): Methamphetamine is a powerful stimulant drug that contains chemicals called amphetamines. Physically, it can have effects on the user similar to cocaine and heroin. It can cause changes in mood, perception, and behavior that range from euphoria to agitation depending on frequency of use and other factors.

Ceremonial tobacco use (legal): Tobacco is indigenous to North and South America and is a member of the nightshade family. Native Americans cultivated tobacco in order to use it as an herbal remedy. They also used it for ceremonial purposes. The Spanish brought it back to Europe in the 1500s, and it then became popular worldwide. In the United States, tobacco was used both by colonists and soldiers during the Revolutionary War. Today, it is often smoked in cigarettes, cigars, pipes, or water pipes called hookahs.

Heroin (illegal): Heroin is an opioid drug that comes from morphine, a natural substance extracted from certain varieties of poppy plants. A person may inject, sniff, swallow, or smoke heroin to experience intense euphoria and relaxation. It can also suppress pain and relieve coughs due to colds or other respiratory illnesses.

Methadone (illegal): Methadone is a synthetic opioid that is used in the treatment of heroin addiction. It blocks the effect of heroin, allowing a person to stop using it while reducing painful withdrawal symptoms.

Lysergic acid diethylamide (illegal): LSD was first synthesized in 1938 by Albert Hofman, a chemist working for Sandoz Laboratories in Basel, Switzerland. It is a hallucinogenic drug that disrupts coordination and produces hallucinations. LSD produces a psychedelic experience, making people feel detached from their bodies, seeing and hearing things that are not really there. It is very addictive.

These drugs all have extremely serious side effects if used in large doses. They may be highly addictive and have serious, long-term health consequences. Research made by the National Institute on Drug Abuse suggests that people who use these drugs are more probably to commit crimes than other people, including violent crimes like armed robbery.

Most of these drugs are illegal and have been for decades, but some are legal for therapeutic purposes such as nicotine and caffeine.

2

LEGAL CLASSIFICATION OF DRUGS BASED ON THEIR RISK POTENTIAL

The government has classified drugs to indicate the level of risk they pose to individuals. This classification is the most significant difference between legal drugs and illegal drugs. Possession, distribution, or use of a drug which has not been approved for medical purposes is illegal. This applies to cocaine, heroin, and marijuana too.

A national survey that was conducted in the United States indicates that 20 percent of US adults have tried illegal drugs at least once in their lifetime. The majority of the users are young adults, and the number continues to increase year after year. The most regularly used drug is marijuana, followed by heroin, cocaine, methamphetamines, ecstacy and inhalants.

From a historical perspective, the use of illegal drugs was prevalent before the 20th century. Cocaine was derived from the cocoa plant and was most commonly used as a substitute for alcohol during that time. These days, the drug has been substituted by psychotropic drugs, such as methamphetamine (crank) or cocaine derivatives.

The government has come up with a list of accepted drugs; these have been proven to have medicinal value. Drugs that have been included in this list, but are used excessively and possess the potential for abuse, have been classified as controlled substances. Examples of such controlled substances include morphine, cocaine, and amphetamines. These are given special attention since they are addictive and cause potential harm to the individual.

Addictive drugs can be classified based on their chemical structure or pharmacological properties. Drug classification can be based on the drugs at issue, the distribution of drugs, or the harms caused by drugs.

Drugs may also be classified and classified based on their harmful effects and their level of risk to society. The classification process is a science that relates to the understanding of how a certain type of drug is produced, transported (by people or commodities), used, sold, and abused. Major drug types are considered under four major levels: A through D.

It is important to note that legalization of drugs does not eliminate the problem of drug abuse; rather, it can even increase it. Legalization means that the distribution or trade of a certain drug is allowed. The word 'legalization' does not mean 'regulation'. The law gives the state the authority to regulate and control the manufacture, sale, and use of a drug within its borders; this way, it maintains order in society. Drugs such as morphine may be sold legally with prescriptions in some countries. While cocaine and marijuana may be illegal, they are sold legally in regulated doses. Some use marijuana for medicinal purposes and some use it recreationally.

Classification is a key to the administration of drug laws. Without any classification, it would be extremely difficult to enforce laws against drug distribution and sales; therefore, it would be impossible to control the scope of drug usage in the country. Classification puts in place regulations on the purchase and sale of drugs so that they can be properly monitored.

To combat drug abuse and addiction, some countries have taken the initiative to stop the international production of narcotics such as opium poppy, coca and cannabis. They have also enacted policies that limit and control the consumption of drugs in their own country. But no matter how well-intended these policies may be, they are still not enough to reduce the prevalence of drug abuse. This is because drug use is a social issue, not a legal one.

The government can control and regulate the sale and use of certain types of drugs such as morphine or cocaine. But as for other types of drugs that are not easily regulated, the best way to stop its spread is for people to be informed about substance abuse and the potential danger it brings with it. And if an individual decides on his or her own volition to try out a drug, he or she should at least know how addictive it may be.

The widely held belief that drug use is a personal issue that should not concern the government is simply wrong. Statistics from the US indicate that substance abuse can lead to a number of social issues such as increased crime rates, a high rate of teenage pregnancy, and an increase in sexually transmitted diseases. Drug abuse is clearly a problem that cannot be ignored. The government plays an important role in addressing this problem by providing lots of information to the public about drugs and how they should be used responsibly.

FIVE CATEGORIES OF DRUGS (FROM MOST TO LEAST RISK)

There are five categories of drugs that are widely used, abused, and produce a major effect on the human body. Some drugs can be of assistance to a person's life, while others might result in death or serious harm.

The most popular drugs that fall under this category are alcohol, tobacco/nicotine, other prescription and over-the-counter medications, recreational drugs, marijuana, and anabolic steroids.

A drug is considered as a schedule I drug if it is recognized as dangerous with no currently accepted medical use in treatment. An illicit drug in its pure form is classified as a schedule I drug. Examples include heroin and LSD.

A drug is classified as a schedule II if it has a high potential of abuse, has previously accepted medical use with severe restrictions, and if the abuse of the drug may lead to severe psychological or physical dependence. An example of a schedule II drug is cocaine.

A drug is classified as a schedule III if it has medical use but abuse can lead the way to moderate or low physical dependence or high psychological dependence. Examples of schedule III drugs are morphine, codeine, and oxycodone.

A drug is classified as a schedule IV if it has mild toxic properties, moderate medical use, moderate potential for abuse relative to other schedules, and less severe withdrawal symptoms than other schedules. Examples of schedule IV drugs include anabolic steroids and cyclazocine.

A drug is classified as a schedule V if it has low potential for physical or psychological dependence relative to other schedules and can be used without a prescription, but may still lead to psychological and physical dependence. Examples of schedule V drugs include Benadryl, ambenonium, atropine, codeine, hydrocodone, phenylephrine, phenyfenoxamine (diphenhydramine), and pseudoephedrine.

Some of the criteria used to determine if a drug will fall into one of the above categories are:

Intended users

A substance can only be scheduled if the drug is intended for unlawful use (e.g. production would not be necessary).

Prevalence in the community

The prevalence of use, illicit or otherwise, must be sufficient to warrant control.

The prevalence of drug use is usually measured by the number of individuals within the population that have ever used. For example, cannabis has a high prevalence due to its widespread and historical use throughout the world.

The level of prevalence is also often relative to the number of individuals who are expected to be users at any given time (often referred to as "at risk" population). The "at risk" population is obtained from the general population (e.g. individuals aged 14 and over).

The prevalence of at-risk populations is usually measured in terms of "one-off" uses. This means that if a drug is present in an individual's possession, then it can be reasonably assumed that the individual has used or intends to use some quantity of the drug. This does not mean that the concerned person has used recently, or on a regular basis (e.g. daily).

Level of harm

The degree of harm is determined by the "medical, social and legal consequences (of use)".

A combination of various factors are considered when determining the level of harm a drug poses. Some examples include:

Type and degree of physical dependence

The level of tolerance within an individual can determine how easily he or she becomes physically dependent on a given substance. The level of tolerance develops based on repeated use within an individual, and thus often depends on the type/frequency used.

The availability of more harmful substances

Certain drugs are prohibited or controlled, meaning they are highly restricted. The substances that are available to the individual must be sufficiently similar/substantially less harmful than the prohibited drug.

Research on Cannabis in particular has shown that the amount of harm/pleasureable effects change based on: If a person is highly tolerant or dependent, he/she will get a greater feeling of euphoria from using larger doses than someone without such tolerance or dependence.

Also, research has shown that the dose that causes the "high" will be slightly different for each person. This is due to variation in biological and psychological factors. For example, individual differences can influence how desirable a given drug is (which has also been termed as a "pleasure-seeking propensity"). Using a drug in moderation can make it more pleasurable, and increase the likelihood of addiction. Also, psychological factors such as cognitive factors (e.g. perception of the drug, effects of the drug), as well as environmental factors such as stress and social factors (e.g. peer pressure) can influence how pleasurable a given drug is to a person.

The mental and physical health condition of the user

The user's mental and physical health can determine the level of harm the drug poses to him/her. For instance, it is important to distinguish between physical dependence (physical symptoms that occur when stopping drug use) and psychological dependence (the feeling that one cannot function without using a given drug).

One clear distinction is that physiological dependence does not require a psychological addiction, although there can be cases where an individual is psychologically addicted to a substance without being physically dependent.

The potential for abuse

The potential for abuse of a drug is based on how easy it is to create the dependence, and how difficult it is to get off of the substance. The best example of this idea is nicotine. Nicotine is very easy to become dependent on (low difficulty), but also has very high levels of physical dependence (high difficulty).

Important Note: There are some drugs for which the difficulty rating provided above does not accurately reflect their ease/difficulty in getting off of them. This is because some drugs are self-administered (e.g. Nicotine) or very difficult to obtain (e.g. heroin), meaning that the potential for dependence/abuse is low even if people with lower mental health may use it and become dependent on it.

In assessing a drug's potential for abuse, physical dependence is not necessarily taken into account, as this relies on factors unrelated to the drug itself; these factors can include tolerance, psychological dependence and abstinence symptoms which are considered in the development of a diagnosis of substance dependence.

ALCOHOL, CANNABIS, COCAINE, OPIATES AND SYNTHETIC DRUGS

The misuse of drugs is a serious health and social problem. In the past, different drugs were treated differently. Alcohol and nicotine were legal, but other drugs such as heroin and cocaine were banned. Today many substances have been declared illegal on a worldwide basis.

Many people misuse alcohol or use drugs as a way of coping with life's problems or to get away from unpleasant feelings. Drugs can make people feel good for a short time because they have an effect on the brain's chemistry. Drug misuse can lead to health problems. The misuse of illicit drugs leads to death through overdose and also severe physical and psychological problems.

Alcohol

Alcohol is the most widely used drug around the world. Alcohol contributes to accidents, crime, assaults and injuries among other things. Drinking can affect a person's ability to think rationally: it may make people feel good or bad and lead them into dangerous situations.

Alcohol is also responsible for many cancers and liver diseases. In England and Wales, it is estimated that about two thirds of the people who die from cancer drink alcohol in excess. Women are statistically more probably to die from cancer because of their drinking habits. Alcohol is also linked with many sexually transmitted diseases including AIDS and the Human Papilloma Virus (HPV). Illegal drug use increases during the winter months when alcohol consumption rises as temperatures drop.

Cannabis (also known as cannabis, marijuana or grass)

Cannabis is a flowering plant which contains a chemical called delta-9-tetrahydrocannabinol (THC). The amount of THC in cannabis varies considerably from drug to drug, but the levels are high enough to produce an intoxicating effect. Presently, there is no way of knowing exactly what dose of THC will be effective for different people.

Cannabis is usually smoked, but it may also be taken as a liquid or by mouth. It is sometimes mixed with tobacco.

Cannabis impairs co-ordination and affects perception, mood and judgement. By interfering with the memory center of the brain, it can produce impaired memory for short periods of time. There are a variety of psychological side effects associated with its use including panic, paranoia and thoughts of suicide. Some people have reported seeing colors more intensely while using cannabis.

Cocaine

This is a stimulant drug derived from the coca plant. It is usually found in the form of cocaine hydrochloride, which is a white powder. It can be sniffed, injected or smoked. Cocaine acts on the brain by blocking its chemical messages; this results in higher concentrations of dopamine – a chemical substance that transmits nerve signals - in specific areas of the brain. Dopamine is linked with feelings of pleasure and euphoria.

Cocaine can cause many health problems including severe breathing difficulties, heart failure, depression, anxiety and panic attacks. It is also associated to an increased risk of a number of cancers including those of the mouth – the heroin or crack habit can lead to the development of cancerous tumors in the oral cavity - and lung. Cocaine can increase blood pressure in some people, which may result in severe headaches or brain damage. Cocaine addiction is often accompanied by psychosis and paranoia. Chronic use of cocaine can lead to a degenerative brain disease known as chronic cerebellar atrophy.

Cocaine is usually inhaled, injected or snorted. It is also smoked, dissolved in water and taken orally.

Cocaine is often combined with heroin or crack because of its ability to produce a powerful high which lasts between one and three hours. Cocaine use leads to increases in heart rate and blood pressure, which may result in heart attacks and strokes.

Opiates

Opiates are drugs that contain opium. Opiate drugs include heroin, morphine and codeine. Addiction to these drugs is a concern for society with devastating consequences for the individual. The opiates interact with the brain's chemical messengers, called neurotransmitters, in such a way that causes changes in mood and state of consciousness. These changes are perceived as pleasurable by the user. This is the reason why people use opiate drugs – for instance heroin – and become addicted to them.

Synthetic drugs

Synthetic drugs are manufactured in a laboratory and come in many forms such as powders, pills, liquids, crystals or a combination of several forms. They are usually sold as 'legal highs' and have been designed to mimic the effects of narcotics such as amphetamines and opiates.

Synthetic drugs are unpredictable substances that vary greatly in their effects. The substances include amphetamines like: 2C-B, ecstasy (MDMA) and GHB. These drugs produce hallucinogenic effects similar to those of LSD. The mental symptoms of these drugs are severe anxiety and paranoia.

Synthetic drugs are also called 'designer drugs' because they are manufactured in laboratories and can be chemically engineered to produce a new substance that is completely different from the one it was originally designed to mimic. The reality that most of these substances have never been tested on humans makes their effects even more unpredictable.

3

HOW DOES DRUG ABUSE AFFECT HEALTH?

There are several areas of human health that are affected by drug abuse, including: physical, mental, social and behavioral. For example, drugs can cause over-stimulation of the central nervous system which can lead to heightened anxiety or even psychotic episodes. Aside from these effects on the brain and body, drug abuse also has an influence on behavior. For example many people who have used drugs have difficulty forming healthy relationships with others because they don't trust them or feel as though they cannot be trusted in return due to past experiences and habits.

While chronic or long-term drug abuse can have a significant impact on the human body and may cause serious health problems, it's important to remember that drug abuse is a complex issue that affects each person differently. Therefore, the specific effects of drug abuse vary depending on the individual as well as the type of drug used and over what period of time it was used. For example, someone who uses drugs occasionally may not suffer from any noticeable ill effects on their health or appearance while someone else who uses the same type of drugs with greater frequency may suffer from severe negative physical or mental side effects.

In addition to causing other health problems and the risk of developing an addiction, drug abuse can also cause other unwanted and unintentional changes in behavior. For example, some people who abuse drugs may begin to smoke or take illegal prescription drugs that do not have any potential for causing damage to the body.

When people use drugs, they often have an intention of altering their state of mind or body as a means to relieve some pain, or to satisfy some emotional need. For example, addicts may smoke marijuana because it makes them feel "high," which in turn deadens their anxiety and helps them take the edge off. However, drug use has negative effects on the person's health and well-being. The people most susceptible to drug abuse are young men in their early twenties. Mental health plays a huge part in drug abuse and addiction. It is important to work on your mental health as well as physical health when it comes to drug and alcohol abuse.

MEDICAL CONSEQUENCES OF DRUG USE

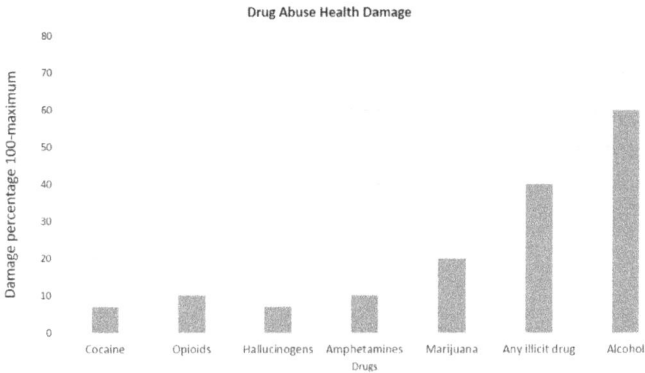

Drug Abuse Health Damage

Drugs do carry some medical consequences. The side effects of drugs are not usually a problem once the drug has been stopped, but they still occur for some users long after they have stopped taking the drug. For example, a cough can be from smoking marijuana or crack cocaine. It is also possible to develop a needle track abscess from drug use. These abscesses can become infected, in which case they are called septicemia.

Users of drugs like crystal meth abuse their bodies adversely by using toxic chemicals that cause so much damage to the body that it will not recover fully or at all. The result is often irreversible damage, leaving individuals with severe irreversible disabilities such as brain damage and memory loss, and often resulting in death.

Drugs not only have immediate consequences, but they also can be expected to have negative consequences in the future. For instance, studies have shown that people who use drugs are more likely to commit violent crimes. As an outcome, the rate of drug-induced deaths has increased dramatically since the early 1980s.

Another medical concern is addiction. It is very common for people to become addicted to drugs and unable to stop using them even though they become addicted to them or even when they are no longer getting high from the drug. Some people are addicted to drugs that are psychologically addictive, such as caffeine or nicotine, instead of physically addictive drugs. Some addiction occurs from using a drug to get a desired effect without the actual high. This can occur with opiates, such as heroin, and stimulants, such as cocaine.

Other adverse consequences from drug use can be made worse by multiple drug use. The combination of two or more drugs can lead to an overdose that can cause death. An overdose can also cause one drug to have a more serious effect than it would have otherwise. An overdose on drugs, or even just giving more than the recommended amount of a drug, will cause a person to become very ill. A common problem involves people injecting too much of a drug and damaging their veins (drug vein syndrome). This will lead to more serious problems like blood clots in the legs.

Other adverse effects from drugs include sudden unexpected death syndrome, also known as SUD or SUDS for short. This can occur when someone has consumed a drug in a very large amount. These deaths are often referred to as "accidental overdoses" or "excess suicides". In these cases, the person likely did not realize that they had taken an overdose of the drug until it was too late for them to stop taking it. This can happen accidentally or by accident if someone overdoses and falls asleep due to using a sedative-hypnotic.

Another serious problem is synthetic drug use. These occur when people create a new drug, often by modifying another drug so that it has a different effect. These are very dangerous, even if they are used in smaller amounts, because users do not know exactly what they are taking. They can be extremely toxic and even fatal to those who use them.

Drug abuse results in many social consequences. Most often, consequences are direct results of the drug use and drug taking activities themselves, such as arrest for possession or sale of drugs. Other times, they arise from the individual's behavior when using drugs, such as reckless driving or engaging in risky sexual behavior. Some consequences are less obvious but no less serious, like development of a tolerance to all other drugs (i.e., "cross-tolerance").

Other consequences involve broader society. These consequences result from actions associated with illicit drug activity, such as money laundering or corruption. Advocates of the drug legalization point out that many of these problems are a result of the illegal status of certain drugs, rather than their pharmacology.

Many negative consequences can occur when someone is using illegal drugs. The side effects of taking illegal drugs vary widely but are usually very dangerous to the individual's health. Many of the side effects are far more severe than the few possible benefits of drug use.

EFFECTS ON THE BRAIN AND BODY

There are many physical and mental effects of drug abuse, the two most common being dependence and withdrawal. The drugs alter the brain's natural chemistry, which can lead to addiction. Research has shown that drug use changes the brain in many ways, altering the ability for people to make decisions. Drug abuse changes the manner a person thinks, feels, behaves and reacts to situations. In addition to these effects on the mind, drugs can have a profound effect on a person's body as well. Drugs are chemicals that can cause changes in the way the brain works. Once a person abuses drugs, he or she may experience many uncomfortable symptoms.

Effects on the Body

Drugs have physical effects on the body in almost every area of the body. After taking drugs, some people experience many unpleasant physical symptoms, such as increased heart rate or blood pressure. Others experience nausea, loss of appetite, sweating, and shaking. In addition to these physical symptoms, drug abuse can cause users to have decreased coordination or tremors. Drug abuse also makes it harder for a person's body to fight diseases or infections. Most drugs have effects on the body beyond that of a normal reaction to a foreign substance or chemical. Drugs are usually more dangerous than other types of chemicals because their effects do not wear off when the chemical is no longer used by the body.

When a person takes illegal drugs, the body may react to them by changing its natural ability to react to pain. This can result in barbiturates or opiates that can make an addict's tolerance for pain increase over time. People with an altered response to pain may take more drugs than they would like and be unable to feel the effects of the drug after a while. This is one reason why some addicts take increasingly higher doses of drugs when they cannot achieve the desired effect. This can result in sickness and organ damage.

Once withdrawal from the drug begins, the body takes it as a sign that it needs more of the drug to make itself feel good. When a person stops taking drugs, the body can become extremely uncomfortable. The most usual pain is in the muscles that control breathing. The effects of withdrawal are intense cravings and strong motivation to take drugs. It is also very possible for people to have withdrawal symptoms when they stop using methadone or other medications as well. The most common ones are extreme restlessness, sweating, nausea and vomiting. Withdrawal can also cause muscle pain and weakness.

Effects on the Brain

Drug abuse affects the brain, especially the areas that control memory, emotions and pleasure. The drugs also affect the areas of the brain responsible for attention and learning. Repeated use of drugs eventually leads to changes in these areas, making it more difficult for people to control their drug use. Over time, the drugs can alter the way a person thinks and feels.

One area affected by drug abuse is memory. When a person takes drugs, it is absorbed into their bloodstream and carried throughout their body. Different drugs affect different parts of our brain and many of them cross into other areas as well. The chemicals found in drugs can actually destroy brain cells, especially in the areas of memory and learning. This leads to memory problems and a higher risk of developing Alzheimer's disease later in life.

Studies show that certain drugs can damage the brain's pleasure center and the frontal cortex. The pleasure center is responsible for producing feelings of happiness, but drug abuse may prevent people from feeling satisfied with normal activities or experiences. The frontal cortex controls impulses, so people who abuse drugs may have a hard time controlling their behaviors because it is damaged by drug use.

Many studies have shown that the brain is still developing in teenagers and that drug abuse can cause permanent changes in their brain. The teenage brain is still growing, so drugs can cause these changes to occur faster than they would otherwise. Some of the changes that can be caused by drug abuse include cognitive development, areas related to attention and memory problems. It is possible for a person's IQ to become permanently lower if he or she abuses drugs at a young age because their brains will not develop as normally as they could have.

The brain is a complex organ, and drugs can affect it in many ways. When a person uses drugs, he or she may have problems concentrating and making decisions. People who abuse drugs often suffer from chemical imbalances when they are under the influence of the drug and may have trouble distinguishing between different types of information. They may also become irritable and angry when they do not feel as good as they think they should. If a person abuses drugs over a long period of time, his or her brain chemistry becomes out of balance and it may be hard to feel normal without drugs.

When people stop taking drugs, they may experience physical and mental withdrawal symptoms. During withdrawal, the brain is deprived of the drug that it has come to depend on. The brain reacts by trying to return to its normal state as quickly as possible. This means that the person may feel extremely uncomfortable because all of the symptoms are trying to occur at once. Symptoms of withdrawal from drugs include sweating, nausea, vomiting, cramping and chills. Some people have a hard time staying asleep during the withdrawal period because their brains are still in the process of trying to return to normal.

When people stop using drugs, they may become extremely distressed because of the changes in their brain chemistry. They may also have physical symptoms that are related to these chemical changes. When people become addicted to drugs, they may suffer from depression, lack of sleep or irritability. They may experience a lot of stress and anxiety and feel very anxious when they do not have access to their drug. The person's mood may also change, and he or she may become emotionally unstable. People who stop using drugs may also have problems with their behavior. They may become impulsive or aggressive for no reason and they may not be able to control their behavior at all.

EFFECTS ON CIRCULATORY SYSTEM AND RESPIRATORY SYSTEM

Essentially, drug abuse can cause damage to your circulatory system and respiratory system in various ways. The heart is put under a lot of stress when you take drugs because there is an increased workload on it as the body tries to cope with the substances. The heart muscle can go into an abnormal state and even fail. The irregular rhythm of the heartbeat can be fatal if not treated on time. The blood pressure can also be affected by drugs forcing the heart to work harder. As the drug abuse continues, there is a weakening of the heart muscles and blood vessels which increases chances of developing high blood pressure and other related ailments such as strokes or heart attacks. The lungs have their own problems caused by drug abuse with chronic coughing becoming common as well as the development of pulmonary infections like Tuberculosis among others. If the drug abuse is not cured, the lungs can be permanently damaged. The skin of the body can suffer permanent damage from cracked and bleeding skin, even if you stop taking drugs. The organs themselves can also be damaged and the skin becomes more vulnerable to infections. The brain too is affected by drugs abuse especially if the drugs are injected as this opens up a direct route to the blood stream. The drug abuse causes memory loss for instance and there is possibility of mental illness such as depression or schizophrenia.

4

WHAT CAUSES DRUG ABUSE?

Drug abuse is a complex issue that the different people, institutions and society are struggling with. There are various factors that determine what leads to drug abuse. Some of these factors include genetics, environment, and social economic status. Treatment programs often fail when they only focus on one of these external factors but do not address what leads to the addiction itself.

Typically, drug users have something that triggers their addiction. Most often this trigger is a substance but it can also be emotional factors and experiences. The drug user often uses the drug to treat these triggers and then continues to use the drug because of how it helps them function in certain situations.

Traumatic experiences like parental abandonment or sexual abuse can also lead to drug addiction. The user may attempt to self-medicate in order to fix the emotional pain caused by these experiences and then takes the drug for future situations. Many addicts have a history of attempts to quit using drugs, but they are unsuccessful.

Genetics are a large factor in drug addiction because the two main reasons for addiction are drug dependence and drug tolerance. Addiction studies have found that genetics play a large role because it can influence the susceptibility of children who have parents with an addiction to drugs, which then leads to addiction in the child as well.

Environment can have a large impact on drug addiction. Certain environmental conditions can lead to the user developing an addiction. Some of these conditions include poverty and social disadvantage. Studies have shown that living in an environment that has a lot of violence can influence the likelihood of drug and alcohol use. Experiences like being the victim of violence can also lead to addiction because the user feels like they need the drug to feel safe in their current situations. The drugs are used as a way for them to cope with the trauma.

The social economic status of a person also plays a role in drug addiction. Negative experiences that come from being poor, do not have good role models, and do not have good overall support can lead to drug addiction. Peer influences can also play a significant role in the development of an addiction. Peer pressure can convince users to take drugs because they see other users doing it which causes them to think that they will lose their friends if they do not use drugs themselves.

Drug abuse is not only something that is determined by these factors, but it is also something that is influenced by the cultural and economic values as well. Substance abuse can lead to substance dependence which can then lead to pathological patterns of use. People who are poor and living in a disadvantaged community are more likely to use a drug due to the fact that they see other users using drugs and they do not see any positive alternatives. Some cultures have better coping methods than others, and even within cultures, there are generational differences. These factors can influence how someone processes stressors and how they deal with their emotions.

The factors that are discussed here can play a significant role in the development of an addiction. The drugs themselves can also cause physical and mental changes which then triggers the user to continue using more and more. Drug use leads to different physical and emotional changes that most people do not notice until it is too late.

The drug user develops a tolerance for the substance and needs to use it more and more to feel the same effects. The drug user then has no other option besides using the substance to feel happy and calm. Soon after continuing their use of the drug, they develop a new habit that is often hard to break.

The user develops physical dependence on the substance and needs the drug in order to function normally. They start to feel worse without the drug and will then turn to it again in order to feel good.

The user may also develop psychological dependence on the drug. The psychological dependence is a mental addiction that develops in the users mind. They will do just about anything to use the drug and they refuse to stop using it no matter what the consequences are.

The user may begin to feel like they need the drug to make it through life without kicking them into depression or an emotional breakdown. Many times, many users continue taking drugs even after knowing that they are causing harm to other people or themselves. They do not care how the drug affects their life or the lives of others because they have become so emotionally and physically dependent on it.

The user commits crimes to get money for drugs when they run out of their supply. They may also steal things from others to sell so that they can have more money to buy their next hit. The user may steal from family members, friends, co-workers and even strangers. They will do anything to get more drugs in their system; this is usually due to the physical addiction they have developed.

CHEMICAL BIOLOGY OF ADDICTION

Drug abuse, or drug addiction, is the compulsive use of a psychoactive substance despite adverse consequences. Broadly speaking, drug addiction may refer to an addiction to chemical substances such as opioids, cocaine, stimulants, barbiturates, and cannabis. Drug addiction is not a single disorder but rather a group of behavioral disorders involving compulsive drug-seeking and use despite harmful consequences. One can be addicted to drugs like opium, heroin, alcohol and tobacco in different ways. Addiction to certain drugs may be more problematical than others in that the addict is driven by a compulsive urge to use the substance; the consequences of continued usage are overwhelming and prompt his willing surrender of self-control.

Most addictions are classified as "tolerance" disorders. The more of any drug a person consumes, the less effective it becomes for achieving an effect. While the user continues to use the substance, less of it is required to achieve the same result. Tolerance usually develops to a substance at first usage or with repeated use. Tolerance is not absolute and varies by substance. For example, tolerance is often developed to caffeine (a stimulant) but not nicotine (a depressant). A person that is experienced with an addictive drug of any type may be able to use or abuse the same amount yet achieve greater effect. Most people develop tolerance by using the drug on a daily basis, but some may build it up quickly through only occasional use. The best method to prevent tolerance is to only use the drug on a "as needed" basis and stopping abruptly when it no longer achieves desired results.

A small amount of any substance that causes a high can have desirable effects, such as counteracting drowsiness caused by another substance, such as alcohol or some types of depressants. A tolerance to these substances can develop. However, it is highly unlikely that the euphoria of a small amount of any drug would be sufficient to cause addiction. Some drugs, such as nicotine can cause a person to become physiologically dependent on the drug after short-term use. This is known as "nicotine withdrawal". Once dependence has occurred, people may have cravings for the drug and also desire more of it in order to prevent withdrawal effects; they begin using their drug more often and in larger amounts than before. Dependence in stimulants such as cocaine and amphetamine often results in a person becoming paranoid, anxious, or withdrawn. A person experiencing this type of drug dependence may feel like they need to continue to use the drug just to feel normal.

Many people who are addicted to drugs or alcohol also suffer from other kinds of mental illness. Among those who are addicted, there are high levels of anxiety, depression, and antisocial personality disorder. These disorders typically begin before drug abuse does, suggesting that the drug is a coping mechanism for these problems rather than the cause.

Drug Addiction (as well as any addiction) is a brain disease. It changes how the brain regulates thoughts, emotions and behaviors. In order to function normally, the brain needs a healthy chemical balance. It is the brain's way of regulating itself. When someone is addicted to drugs, his or her body gets used to having the drug in it. This leads to physical dependence and compulsive drug seeking behavior. If an addict doesn't have access to his or her drug, he or she will usually feel uncomfortable and actually experience withdrawal symptoms if too much time goes by between using their drug of choice. Some withdrawal symptoms are headaches, sweating, tremors, full body pain and vomiting. The addict will often crave their drug of choice and suffer severe psychological distress if they don't get it.

GENETIC PROFILE OF PEOPLE WITH BAD HABITS

It's easy to think of people with bad habits as radically different from you, but the truth is that they probably have a genetic profile just like yours. In fact, research has shown that people who struggle with drug addiction or other types of compulsive behaviors share the same gene variants as those who are predisposed to schizophrenia, depression, and attention deficit disorders.

However, their genes don't make them vulnerable to these problems---their genes merely make them more susceptible to developing these kinds of disorders. That means that people who are struggling with habits and addictions actually have a stronger gene pool than those who don't suffer from these problems.

The question is, why have those gene variants mutated and become problematic? The most likely culprits are environmental stresses---either the family environment or peer group or a combination of the two. Other reasons may include childhood trauma or a bad relationship with a parent. Being around other people with the same genetic problems can also lead to negative habits and behaviors.

It is not that people are genetically predisposed to develop drug problems, but rather that the genetics predispose them to various types of behavior, including drug abuse.

In recent years there has been a great deal of enthusiasm for studying genetic factors in addiction and compulsive disorders. Not only do genes play a powerful role in many physical illnesses, but they also influence emotional and behavioral aspects of an individual's life. Research has shown that our DNA influences our brain chemistry and that our biochemistry changes with age.

In other words, our behavior becomes more entrenched as time goes on. That's why it's so crucial to examine the childhood environment of someone who has a drug abuse problem. If the person was raised in an unstable household and is now struggling with substance abuse, then he or she needs a lot of support from friends and family members who can help him or her find appropriate outlets for frustration and anger that might otherwise lead to addiction.

When people have a genetic predisposition to addiction they're more likely to develop bad habits. There's also a genetic component to compulsive behaviors, which might include gambling, overeating, or other types of negative behaviors. These are called addictive disorders.

It is true that many people with an addictive personality also have a strong desire for sensation and experience, which leads them to dangerous activities. Their genetic makeup leads them to seek intense stimulation, and drug abuse provides that satisfaction. So, for many people, substance abuse is a means of reaching out. They're not really seeking drugs---they just want someone to reach out to them.

GLOBAL DRUG ABUSE

In 2020, 35 million people globally are drug abusers. This is three times the amount that was estimated in 2005. This staggering figure comes from a recent report by the United Nations Office on Drugs and Crime (UNODC). In the report on drug abuse, UNODC provides information about trends in cannabis, amphetamine-type stimulants (ATS), opiates, cocaine and new psychoactive substances (NPS).

According to the report, drug abuse has indeed reached a crisis level in North America. The drug abuse problem is especially severe in the US where over 14 million people are using illegal drugs. This makes almost 22% of the population of US which is a very large number in comparison to other regions. On an average, every day, an average of 130 people die from drug overdose in America. Another shocking statistic is that one out of every three children end up using drugs before they hit 18 years old.

In Europe, drug abuse has reached critical levels in countries like UK, Netherlands and Germany. The report suggests that over 3 million Europeans use opioid drugs. In fact, it is estimated that 50% of Europe's heroin users live in the UK.

The report also details drug abuse trends in Asia. In Japan, drug abuse mainly involves methamphetamine or crystal meth. Other regions such as Indonesia and China are also facing high level of drug abuse. In fact, in some Asian societies like Thailand the use of meth has increased up to 250%.

The report also mentions that in Africa, there is a significant increase in drug abuse cases especially for heroin and ATS. The report states that three million African youths are addicted to drugs with most of them being addicted to opiates.

The report further states that many new psychoactive substances are being used in the world and they are increasing at an alarming rate and becoming a threat to public health.

According to the estimate, drug abuse is a major public health challenge. Therefore, there is need for countries to work together to fight this problem. However, this is not an easy task as the problem is global and affects the whole world.

According to UNODC, drug abuse and addiction can be prevented by addressing prevention, treatment and rehabilitation through policies that address risk and protective factors. Furthermore, countries must provide support for people with drug abuse problems who want to seek help rather than shun them. In addition to this, family members of those suffering from drug abuse need to understand that they are not responsible for this problem and they should provide support rather than blame the victim.

However, it is also necessary to realize that people are different and therefore different approaches should also be employed in dealing with drug abuse.

In the report, UNODC suggests that all countries should have comprehensive drug policies which include prevention, treatment and rehabilitation programs. The aim of these programs is to reduce the related harms by preventing the situation from developing into a problem at all.

UNODC recommends a number of measures such as producing more information about key issues surrounding drug abuse and reducing stigma associated with it. In addition, these programs should address the causes of drug abuse and improve the health and social outcome.

The report also calls for measures which promote harm reduction. Harm reduction involves reducing the negative consequences of drug use through policy interventions. Furthermore, programs should be integrated with other strategies as well as services to prevent drug abuse and reduce the related harms.

5

THE LEGAL AND SOCIETAL
IMPLICATIONS OF DRUG ABUSE

Drug abuse is a modern day epidemic that has reached new heights in recent years. Once a problem largely confined to social circles, drug abuse has now become prevalent across the globe with an estimated 120 million people using drugs in some form.

In addition to causing physiological harm, drug abuse also carries significant legal and societal implications. The various facets of this issue are examined below.

Societal Implications of Drug Abuse

Society as a whole is affected by the negative consequences that stem from drug use. These individuals do things they otherwise would not do when under the influence of drugs, and these actions can have ramifications for society as a whole. An example of the societal impact resulting directly from drug abuse could be seen in a case recently reported in New York City, where a woman used crack cocaine and subsequently set her apartment on fire while under the influence (Goldstein). With the drug use, the woman was essentially impaired and unable to distinguish between reality and fantasy. Further, because of the euphoric effect of drugs, the individual may feel invulnerable or impervious to negative consequences. The societal implications resulting from this type of behavior are potentially devastating. Drug users could cause harm to others through reckless or random actions and/or neglectful behavior that can lead to injury or even death.

The existence of drug users also has a deleterious effect on society as a whole. The individuals who use drugs are not typically the most productive, law-abiding members of society. To the contrary, these individuals are often unreliable in their duties and responsibilities and can become a burden to the rest of society. Alternatively, drug users could potentially be productive members of society if their drug abuse was curbed or eliminated. As one agency states, "the effects that drugs have on a person's ability to be productive cannot be ignored" (National Institute on Drug Abuse).

Legal Implications of Drug Abuse

Drug abuse can have many adverse legal consequences. Although the use of many different substances is banned, just about any substance used for recreational purposes is considered to be illicit. If someone is caught with drugs, they are subject to both criminal and civil sanctions, depending on the type of drug in question. If an individual is convicted for drug possession, they could face jail time or a fine. Obviously, if someone is caught selling or distributing drugs, they are subject to harsher legal consequences than a person who was caught with the substance for personal use. If any minors are involved in drug related activity, they and their parents could face stiff penalties for the involvement of the minor in criminal acts.

The introduction of drugs into society has had a profound impact on the legal system. The use of drugs in criminal trials is rising dramatically, and most states have altered their statutes to account for this trend. In addition, society has also been adversely affected by the rise in drug use. With more people using drugs, there are more people abusing substances and committing crimes.

In addition to the legal ramifications of using drugs, the societal implications of drug abuse have a strong negative effect on the family structure. Those people who are under the influence of drugs can be a detriment to family life and could lead to the breakdown of families. Additionally, children who have parents who are addicted to drugs may be subject to abuse through their parents.

Society has grown increasingly concerned with drug abuse in recent years because of its effects on society as a whole. Although many individuals use drugs for recreation purposes and do not experience any negative consequences, they can be a detriment to society at large.

The legal and societal implications of drug abuse are numerous and complex. The issue of drug abuse is one that must be addressed universally. This does not imply a forced or heavy-handed solution to the problem, but rather the implementation of programs and services designed to help those suffering from drug abuse problems.

EFFECTS ON THE COMMUNITY

Drug abuse has many negative effects on the community. One negative effect is that drugs can cause crime. For example, drug crimes create theft and violence. A person who is addicted to drugs may commit a crime in order to buy drugs.

A second negative effect of drug abuse on the community is addiction, which can also lead to family problems and poverty. Addiction can lead people who are addicted to stop caring about other people, including their children or spouse. People who are addicted may not want to work and may lose their job. Drug use can lead some addicts into criminal behavior, such as theft and prostitution. This is because an addict will do anything to get drugs.

A third negative effect of drug abuse on the community is a decline in the quality of life. Drug addicts may use their time to get drugs instead of doing activities that are socially important, like family time or volunteering for a good cause. The people around them notice this and may not want to be with them.

A fourth negative effect of drug abuse on the community is that it can make an individual or a group of people violent. It causes people to act aggressively. If someone is addicted, they will do anything they can to get drugs. They may use bad techniques to get drugs, such as robbing a store or stealing from an individual. Some people become very violent if they are addicted because they do not want anyone to stop them from getting drugs.

Drug abuse is becoming more and more popular. It is a serious problem for kids, teens, young adults and families in every community. Drug abuse can be a big threat to the community because people who are addicted may not work or take care of their families. For example, an addiction could lead to poverty. It is important for people and society to stand up against drug abuse. Many agencies are working hard to fight drug abuse and help people who are addicted. We can work together to prevent drug abuse.

EFFECTS ON THE FAMILY STRUCTURE, SEX LIFE AND ECONOMIC STATUS OF PEOPLE

The cost of drug addiction to the family structure, sex life and economic status of people who suffer from it is huge. Here are some ways it affects various members in a family when the one suffering does not receive treatment.

In the family structure, it is responsible for the loss of a father, husband and/or other important men in the household. It makes the woman who doesn't seek treatment feel like she is being judged. It only increases her frustration toward her husband, parents and/or children due to her inability to provide a stable lifestyle for them while she is still under its influence. It has also destroyed relationships between loved ones when their loved one either needs to be hospitalized or incarcerated due to drugs.

Sex life is affected because the addict can't fulfill his sexual needs or desires. It also affects the spouse by due to the rise of STDs and lack of desire for the spouse. It is also among one of the reasons why many men and women cheat on their spouses.

Economic status is affected because the addict is no longer able to provide for their family members, who may take up other jobs in order to provide for themselves and/or their children. It also brings a negative effect on the children when the parent is financially unstable, either due to incarceration or hospitalization.

The cost to the family for various drugs is high and can range from tens of dollars to over a thousand dollars depending on what they take. For those who are addicted to painkillers, it can reach as much as $3000 a month on an average basis. It is also expensive to their health, especially if they do not seek treatment. One's family may have to take up jobs that they originally wanted, because things like rent and bills should be taken care of by the addict due to the decline in their productivity at work. If they are not abstaining from drugs, then their productivity will continue to decline and it will make it hard for the family to make ends meet. These are some of the many ways that drug abuse affects the structure of a family and their ability to provide a stable lifestyle for themselves.

Overall, it has a huge effect on various members of the family structure whether they will be more prone to divorce or not. It only makes things harder for the addict, making things worse because they won't listen to any of their family members who are trying to help.

6

HOW CAN DRUG ABUSE BE TREATED?

There are many different treatments available for drug addiction, but the ultimate goal of any treatment program is to reduce, or completely stop, the use of these substances.

Drug abuse is a difficult problem to manage due its very nature. The person who abuses drugs may not be able to control their urge or desire for them. Some drugs give a false sense of well-being, which causes the user to want to feel that way again and again.

An individual who is using drugs may appear distracted or distant from their family and friends. They may also have abrupt mood swings, and sometimes withdrawal from loved ones can happen.

Drug abuse can be treated or managed in both inpatient and outpatient programs. Both can be very effective, depending on the needs of each individual that is suffering from addiction.

Inpatient programs offer more intense treatment for a longer period of time, however some people need the intensive care that an inpatient program provides in order to recover. Inpatient programs give a safe and secure environment in which the individual can focus solely on their recovery, free of any distractions.

The length of inpatient treatment depends on the needs of the individual. Most often it is between 30 and 90 days for most programs, but some can be as short as three days or may last up to one year or more.

Outpatient treatments are also very effective and should be used in conjunction with an aftercare program. The individual must be monitored and supervised by staff members throughout the day, to make sure they are following their rules and are on track to success.

Aftercare programs should be able to provide many of the same services that inpatient programs provide because of the close interaction between patients and program staff members. Some of them will offer psychiatric treatment as well as treatment for physical conditions. Aftercare programs have a course length somewhere between three months and two years.

Depending on the severity of the drug addiction, some people can rely solely on inpatient treatment while others may need to use both inpatient and outpatient programs.

While there are many different types of drug abuse treatment programs, some of them follow a common goal: to help people recover from their addiction. They also help people strengthen their connection with family and loved ones, so they can rebuild and return to their normal lives.

Many different programs are available for drug addiction today, such as residential, counseling, and outpatient programs. Each of these will have different procedures and treatment methods. The treatment plan must be decided on according to the needs of the individual.

Treatment for drug abuse is necessary for the addicted person to regain control over their life. An addict cannot stop using drugs on their own because they are not in control of their actions. Drug abuse treatment helps people to regain this control by removing them from all drugs and distractions.

Drug addiction treatment is generally very successful if an individual has good support from family and friends, as well as a strong desire to get clean.

Drug abuse treatment programs can also help people develop new skills to cope with everyday problems and stress. This will help them control their urges to commit behaviors associated with abuse of drugs.

NON-MEDICAL TREATMENT FOR DRUG ADDICTION

Treatment for drug abuse is a difficult and complicated process. The most effective treatment methods can take time, patience, commitment, and even ability. Non-medical treatments are not always as effective as medical treatments are. Here are some ways that you can get help for your addiction without a doctor:

Take a class

A drug abuse class is given by a drug treatment center, school, or even your community. Drug abuse classes are also called drug education classes and they usually consist of a series of lectures, films, and group discussions. They can be an important step to help you understand the severity of your addiction and see how it negatively impacts you, your family, and the people around you.

Join a support group

Many people who suffer from addiction find support groups useful for maintaining their sobriety. You can attend meetings that are sponsored by your local AA or NA chapter or a non-profit organization. Sometimes you can even find support groups in your city for drugs of abuse, alcohol, and gambling, among others. By attending these meetings you'll meet people who are going through the same things as you and learn from each other.

Volunteer

Make some volunteer work at your local hospital, soup kitchen, church, or community center. Often times your service will be a chance to meet other people who are suffering from the same problems as you. People who need your help can be very helpful in helping keep you out of trouble and prevent relapse to the point that you'll actually need treatment.

Attend school

Drug rehab schools teach and encourage students to learn about addiction before, during, and after their program. These are essential tools that can be performed by anyone, not just drug dependent individuals. Drug rehabilitation schools also help people learn how to live a clean and healthy lifestyle outside of the program.

Take accountability courses

These classes are designed to help people who've already been through treatment understand how their actions affected their loved ones and others around them. They can also teach users how to manage their addiction without using alcohol or drugs. These courses can greatly reduce the chances of relapse into an addiction.

Create a treatment plan

A treatment plan is a written document you create that outlines your goal, strategies you'll use to reach the goal, and things that will help you overcome the addiction. Having something in writing can help you keep on track with your goals and it will also remind you of the commitment you made to your treatment.

Distract yourself from cravings

The best way to stay away from drugs or alcohol is to create activities that will distract yourself from craving them. Try to find things you love doing, like going to the movies or playing sports, and surround yourself with friends who support your sobriety.

Create a list of pros and cons

The reason someone will remain sober after treatment is when they are committed to living a clean and sober lifestyle. So before you begin treatment you should ask yourself why you want to be sober. That question can help motivate you when times get tough during treatment and afterward.

Create a list of goals

Many people who suffer from addiction do not know why they're addicted. To make a drug and alcohol addiction recovery easier you should create a treatment goals list. This list should include what your goals are for living a sober life. Before you begin treatment, you should also study up on the things that will help keep your addiction at bay, like finding support groups in your area, volunteering at a hospital or soup kitchen, and joining an alumni group for people who have completed drug rehab programs.

Join a 12-step group

The 12-step process is a series of steps you have to follow before you can overcome your addiction. The program allows for the people who suffer from addiction to speak about their drug problem, gain new members for support, and work on recovery. This program is an additional treatment option that is non-medical and can be very effective when combined with medication.

These are just some of the non-medical treatments for drug addiction. You may need to try more than one of them to find the method that works best for you and your situation. Remember, any method you try will be easier if you have a therapist or an addiction counselor who can help guide you through the process.

MEDICATION BASED THERAPY FOR DRUG ABUSE

Trying to quit addiction on your own can be difficult, but the right treatment may be easier than you think. Medication-based therapy is a popular treatment for people living with substance use disorder. This form of therapy offers a number of benefits for those looking to kick their addiction, and it is the most effective type of drug abuse treatment available today. It's also one of the only treatments which has been proven to help recovery rates, meaning that rehab centers are seeing positive results when patients complete this type of therapy.

Medication-based therapy for drug abuse is an effective way for people to kick their addiction. While it is the most effective type of drug abuse treatment available, it can also be one of the most difficult to choose. This is because each medication that will be used must go through extensive research and testing before it can be approved by the Food and Drug Administration (FDA).

Luckily, medication-based therapy is a treatment option that has been proven to be successful. It offers a number of benefits —including a non-medicinal approach to prescription medications and the opportunity to tap into the power of a drug while still working on your addiction—and it has helped many addicts in recovery throughout the years. Medication-based therapy may not be for everyone, but it is an excellent choice for people looking for medical support during their recovery from drug abuse.

Medication-Based Therapy for Drug Abuse Works

While medication-based therapy may sound like a modern treatment, the first anti-craving medications were approved for use in 1990. Consequently, scientists have been working hard to develop more medicines to help people recover from drug abuse. Today, there are five medications that have been approved to treat drug abuse, and they work in different ways.

One type of medication-based therapy that is available for drug abuse is medications to complement psychotherapies. While this may appear like an odd combination, it can be a powerful form of drug abuse treatment. These medications can help people regulate their moods, which can make recovery from drug abuse more manageable. The medications involved in this type of medication-based therapy are commonly prescribed to people living with depression or anxiety disorders.

Another type of medication-based therapy is the treatment of opioid use disorders. This type of drug abuse recovery is a three-part form of treatment that includes counseling, medication, and therapy. The medications used include methadone and buprenorphine, which help people deal with their cravings. These treatments are safe and effective for helping people recover from opioid abuse, but they are only available in certain areas—usually through a clinic or a doctor's office.

The three other types of medications that have been approved to treat drug abuse are stimulants, antidepressants, and α-2 agonists. These medications have shown a lot of promise for helping people recover from their drug abuse and can be options for medication-based therapy. Compared to other types of treatments, medications are a more practical option because they require less work—in some cases, you can get the medication at a pharmacy near you.

There are many reasons why people choose medication-based therapy. This type of drug abuse treatment can serve as a support system for anyone looking to kick their addiction, by providing them with medical support. Unlike other types of treatments, people in medication-based therapy will have the opportunity to tap into the power of a drug while still working on their addiction. This means that they will be able to recover more quickly and get back on the right path while staying under medical supervision.

7

WHAT IS THE SCOPE OF DRUG ABUSE IN TODAY'S SOCIETY?

Criminalization of drug abuse can be seen as one of the most controversial topics in today's society. With the increasing prevalence and severity of drug-related activities, it is increasingly difficult to handle this issue on an individual level–in that sense, criminalizing drug abuse is necessary from a society standpoint. More than 100 million Americans (1 out of every 3) have tried some sort of drug in their lifetime, and more than 10 million have a drug or alcohol problem. In the United States only, there are more than 20 million addicts.

The problem of drug abuse is all-encompassing, as it effects every aspect of life. Nearly 37 million people abuse drugs in the United States, spreading its damage to every single aspect of our society. As a result, drug abuse has become a major problem that affects us all.

In the past, the eradication of drug-related activities was conducted at an individual level; that is, there were organizations designed to help people with their addictions and problems. Now, however, criminalization is necessary in order to handle these problems on a society-wide scale.

The government, the schools, and individual communities have all been trying to establish programs to help curb the drug abuse epidemic. The federal government has tried to implement a barrier between children and drugs. Research has been done to find out the best way to do so. The National Institute on Drug Abuse (NIDA) has found that children are at risk for drug abuse at a much younger age than the general public had previously thought. It once was thought that first time drug use occurred in mid-teens but NIDA found out that almost one third of school-age children have tried an illegal drug by the time they reach the 8th grade.

The solution to this drug-abuse problem can be seen in many different aspects. The first thing that appears to mind is the use of a more individualized approach. There are many organizations that are designed to treat and help drug addicts. These organizations can be found almost anywhere in our society. They can be located in big cities, small towns, suburbs and rural areas.

To be successful in treating drug abuse, however, there should be a major emphasis placed on treatment. The focus should not be on criminalization, but rather on treating drug addicts. Drug addiction is just as difficult to treat as any other form of addiction or mental illness, and like all other illnesses, the best way to handle it is individually.

In order for a drug epidemic to be eradicated, it is necessary that individuals are given a chance at treatment. Punishing the addicts after they have been caught is not enough; rather, there should be a big focus on preventing them from becoming addicts in the first place. There must be a major emphasis placed on educating all aspects of our society about the effects of drug abuse and providing all necessary resources to help them. Drug abuse education should also be required for children, so that they are aware of what effects drugs can have on their lives.

Another aspect of eradicating drug abuse in America would be implementing legislation that makes treatment much more accessible and affordable. Treatment for drug addicts should be available in nearly every area of the country in order for the epidemic to be handled correctly.

Finally, the government should implement laws that make drug abuse more of a lesser crime. So that there is an emphasis on rehabilitation and treatment, rather than criminalization.

THE DIFFERENT CLASSES OF DRUGS THAT CAN BE ABUSED IN TODAY'S SOCIETY

Drug abuse is a serious issue in society to the point where it is being looked at as a public health crisis. In 2016, the

Washington State Department of Social and Health Services issued a press release stating that "drug addiction and related substance use disorders are on pace to kill nearly 250,000 Americans this year." There are many different kinds of drugs that are abused in today's society such as prescription drugs, cocaine, methamphetamine, etc.

I will discuss the different classes of drugs which can be abused in today's society. The first class of drugs that can be abused are prescription drugs. Prescription drug abuse is a very serious issue both inside and outside of the United States. In 2003, it was reported that 79% or more than 1 million people in the United States used prescription drugs for nonmedical purposes at least once in their lifetime. It is commonly known where most people go to get their prescription drugs from such as their local pharmacy or going on the streets to sell illegal drugs such as heroin, cocaine etc. In accordance with the National Survey on Drug Use and Health, nearly 106.6 million Americans (18 years or older) had taken prescription painkillers, tranquilizers or sedatives for non-medical purposes at least once in their lifetime. Drugs such as oxycodon, Xanax etc. were the most commonly abused prescription medications. As claimed by the Substance Abuse and Mental Health Services Administration (SAMHSA), in 2014 there were over 2.6 million emergency room visits related to prescription drug misuse. It is also important to note that when the abuse of prescription drugs is occurring it can lead to numerous health and social issues such as depression, anxiety, poor social skills and worse even death. The second class of drugs that can be abused in today's society are illegal drugs. Illegal drugs include cocaine, methamphetamine, heroin etc. The use of illegal drugs can lead to a lot of health and social issue such as addiction, poverty, poor academic performance at school, etc. According to a study done on drug users in the United States, 45% of people who used cocaine recreationally had lost jobs due to it, and 3.6% had been sent to jail. Another study done on the impact of drug abuse in society showed that approximately 2.8 million people over the course of a year were heavy drug users and they accounted for about 58% of all emergency department visits related to nonmedical use of pharmaceuticals. The last class of drugs that can be abused is alcohol. Alcohol is considered as the most abused substance in America. According to a study conducted on alcohol abuse, 15.1 million adults had an alcohol use disorder in 2013 and 1.4 million adults had a serious alcohol use disorder. It is also important to note that the National Survey on Drug Use and Health conducted a survey which said that 98,000 people die every year from alcohol misuse and those who are under 21 years old have an average of 87,000 emergency department visits each year related to alcohol abuse.

Users of illegal drugs such as heroin and methamphetamine are at a high risk for developing mental illnesses. According to the Substance Abuse Mental Health Services Administration, 75.1 million adults have a substance use disorder and of those, 18.9 million people are classified with a "serious" or "chronic" substance use disorder which leads to severe impairment in social, family, school or work functioning. While these numbers are staggering as it is, SAMHSA found out that only 10% of people with a substance use disorder receive treatment at any point in the year.

THE EFFECTS OF DRUG ABUSE ON SOCIETY.

Drug abuse in the United States has been a major problem since the heroin epidemic of the 1970s. With an estimated 54,000 people dying as a result of drug overdoses in 2017, it is more important than ever to understand how substance use can lead to a number of negative consequences for individuals and society.

Here are some facts about the effects of drug abuse on society:

- Deaths and Injuries. Drug abuse has been linked to two-thirds of sudden unexpected deaths in the United States. According to the National Institute on Drug Abuse (NIDA), drug overdoses are considered an epidemic because they account for more than 200,000 deaths each year. Along with drug overdose, prescription drug abuse is also a serious problem.
- Prescription medications prescribed for pain management often end up being used illicitly as well. While there are many medications that can be used to treat pain, NIDA reports that prescription opioids are the most commonly abused drugs in the United States.

- Interpersonal Violence. Substance use can cause interpersonal violence by impairing judgment, encouraging people to engage in risky behavior and making it difficult to manage everyday stress and conflict. In the United States, drug-related homicides are related to drug trafficking and are most often committed with firearms.

- Drugs for sexual abuse are another concern because using these drugs is associated with a high risk of pregnancy and sexually transmitted diseases.

- Dependency. Many addictive drugs make people feel good initially, but long-term use is associated with the opposite effect. Physical effects of drug use are often followed by psychological and social issues that can lead to addiction.

- The physical effects of drug abuse are health problems such as respiratory infections, heart disease, and sexual dysfunction that can result from long-term drug use. Drug abuse also has social consequences such as criminal behavior that can lead to imprisonment or even death.

- Psychosis and Mental Health Issues. Use of hallucinogenic drugs can lead to psychotic symptoms that make it difficult to tell what is real. Psychotic symptoms include hallucinations, delusions, disordered thinking, and paranoia.

- The use of hallucinogenic drugs can also trigger mental

health issues and cause people to be more vulnerable to schizophrenia.

- Drugs for depression or anxiety are associated with an increase in suicidal thoughts and behaviors as well as suicidal plans and attempts.

- Health Problems for Mothers and Their Babies. Substance abuse during pregnancy can lead to temporary or permanent health issues for the fetus. According to one survey, women who abuse drugs during pregnancy are more likely to have newborns that are small for their age, have low birth weights and mental retardation.

- In addition to physical complications, substance use is linked with a number of health problems in infants exposed in the womb. Newborns born to mothers who abused substances during pregnancy are more likely to have medical issues when compared with babies of mothers who didn't use substances while pregnant.

- Crime. Crimes related to substance abuse have become a public health concern in the United States. Many crimes are committed by people who are under the influence of drugs, and substance abuse is a main factor behind a number of violent crimes.

- Based on the Federal Bureau of Investigation (FBI), drug-related crimes are considered violent because they can lead to violence against other people.

- Drug abuse also can lead to other criminal behavior,

making it a contributing factor to many crimes, including property damage and driving while intoxicated (DWI).

- Other Consequences. Using illicit drugs alone is also associated with homelessness, decreasing the quality of life for people who are released from prison as well as those living on the streets.

EMERGING DRUGS OF ABUSE AND THEIR LEGAL STATUS

Theft, violence, and fraud are just a few of the crimes associated with drug abuse. In recent years, the frequency of these crimes has increased alongside an uptick in the popularity of new drugs.

Many believe that illicit substances get into our communities because there's a large demand for them. However, what stands out to us is that many of these drugs have been created and sold legally by pharmaceutical companies as formularies or prescription medications. The illicit trade in prescription drugs is a booming business that is a faster, easier source of revenue than heroin.

The legal question then becomes, "Are all these drugs harmful to health?" The answer isn't as easy as you may think. Legal and illegal substances are macroscopic and microscopic at the same time, like a poison above the ground and a chemical that makes up the water we drink or on our skin. The same substance can be used for medicinal purposes but also in ways that put people at risk for harm. Pharmaceutical companies produce drugs whose main purpose is to treat health conditions but, in some cases, "side effects" are actually more desirable.

Many drugs are known to cause harm or put users at risk of being harmed. Some of these include alcohol, tobacco, marijuana, heroin and methamphetamines. These are classified as "controlled substances" in the United States because they have a high potential for abuse and dependence). In addition, 70% of illicit active substances are used for their euphoric effects. This percentage has been steadily increasing throughout the past few decades and is expected to grow as more people become addicted to prescription drugs.

Cocaine, heroin and methamphetamine are often called "hard drugs" because they are addictive and dangerous to the brain in addition to being very addictive. In the United States, cocaine is not legal anywhere within its borders, and it is a Schedule II drug. When abused, cocaine can produce euphoria combined with energy and increased alertness.

Drug abuse comes in many forms including drinking alcohol at an early age and using drugs to ease pain or escape negative feelings such as anxiety or depression.

Most people believe that marijuana is the least harmful drug available that is why it is now legal in Canada and many other countries. Marijuana affects the brain more than the heart and lungs when it is smoked or consumed in edible form. The effects of marijuana can be seen with synthetic cannabinoids, which are THC analogs that produce similar feelings of euphoria and relaxation as marijuana but without its side effects.

Synthetic cannabinoids can be produced by creating a chemical from Marijuana, which is then sprayed or dripped onto a leaf to create an actual high. The effects of synthetic cannabinoids resemble marijuana but they have been linked to more severe consequences such as an increased risk of panic attacks, depression, psychosis and delusions. That is why the legalization of marijuana is a matter of debate. Synthetic cannabinoids are not regulated by the government and they can be illegal in some places while legal in others.

Some countries today Marijuana is used for Medical Purposes is not a Harmless Tendency, but it is known to relieve Discomfort and Pain.

8

HOW CAN DRUG ABUSE BE PREVENTED?

Drug Abuse is a very significant matter, and even though it is hard to prevent drug abuse from occurring, there are some ways that you can reduce your risk or help someone else who may be affected by it. Many organizations, communities and individuals have been working together to create prevention campaigns or rehabilitation programs for individuals addicted to drugs.

These are some methods you may use to prevent drug abuse:

- If you have a friend who is abusing drugs, talk to them about your concerns and let them know that there are other ways of dealing with their problem. The first step to helping someone is admitting that they may have a problem. Drug affects the brain, how it works, and how it communicates with other parts of the body.

As a person uses more drugs, their brain becomes less able to make good choices and decisions. This can lead to poor health and the risk of getting into legal trouble. Friends can help you recognize when your drug use is leading to problems in your schoolwork, family life, or relationships with friends or other people who matter to you.

- If you work with kids, see if you can get involved in a prevention program at your school. This can help to educate kids that drugs are bad for them and that it is important to make good decisions. In some schools, there are even programs that allow you to do something more on the side like playing sports. This helps you stay away from being with friends who are abusing drugs when you are not at the school.

- Get involved in community organizations or enroll yourself in anti-drug campaigns in your neighborhood, local high schools or colleges. It is essential that everyone must work together to prevent this kind of situation from happening all over again. This also helps you to become more involved with the community and serve as an example to other young people.

- If you are into sports or have been practicing any sport, you can make use of your skills as a positive role model. When kids see someone they admire doing something good in their life, it gives them a good impression on how they should be practicing their skills and how they should use them for the betterment of themselves and others.

- Educate yourself, so that you know the facts about drug abuse and addiction. This knowledge can help you in avoiding bad relationships and helping others to avoid the same problems. The more you know about drugs, the more likely it is that you will be able to spread the word about drug abuse prevention. Educate yourself so that you can dispel myths and misconceptions about drugs, their effects or the use of illegal substances. Additionally educate yourself on having a healthy lifestyle and how to maintain good health - for your own sake as well as those around you.

- Support recovery programs that treat drug addiction. These programs help individuals addicted to drugs withdraw from their addiction and start new lives without needing drugs to satisfy themselves. This helps them to recover and have a happy life in due course of time.

- Ask parents if they are doing all they can to prevent their children from getting involved in harmful activities like drug abuse. Don't just sit around and then do nothing when your child faces a problem that could be prevented from occurring in the first place.

Make sure they know what is going on in the community and that they are informed about the risks associated with harmful activities such as drug abuse.

- Don't even hesitate to talk to someone if you or someone you know abuses drugs. If you or a loved one is struggling with addiction, don't give up. There are many resources to help you fight addiction and change your life for the better. Contact a helpline or talk to your doctor for advice on how best to access drug abuse care.

- Work or volunteer for an organization which helps people who have addictions to drugs or alcohol. You can help provide a service to people who are less fortunate and have nowhere else to turn for help. Addiction is a very difficult thing to deal with and it is important that you find support from people that are working in the same field as you are.

- If you know that someone is thinking about abusing drugs, you can approach them to express your concern and offer advice. You can do this in person, via letter, or over the phone. You can let them know that you are worried about them and that you are willing to help them in any way possible. This will give them a chance to talk about their drug abuse and work towards reducing it.

- If you cannot prevent drug abuse, at least prevent

yourself from being a victim of it. This is why we have to work together with others. At times, we may feel helpless and unable to do anything but doing something good for others when you can do it. Be supportive of those around you and help them when they need it. Accept their people skills and always remember that they can learn from you as well. If your friends are abusing drugs, try to encourage them to do something about their problem because trying drugs does not solve anything.

While it is impossible to completely prevent drug abuse from occurring, there are things that you can do to help yourself and others avoid the dangers of drug abuse.

You can protect yourself and others by learning as much as possible about drugs, how they affect people and what the risks are of abusing them. This way, you can spread the word and help others to avoid getting into trouble.

You can also reduce the chances of being put in a situation where you may have to deal with someone who is high on drugs or has overdosed.

If you see your friends abusing drugs and drinking, let them know that their behavior is unacceptable and that they need to stop. Share your thoughts and concerns with them. Explain the dangers of drug abuse to them and how it can affect their health in the future if they continue using these substances.

If you or someone you know is abusing drugs, seek help immediately. Drug abuse is not a joke and there are serious consequences of using these substances. If you do not get help, your life could end as a result of drug addiction.

MEANS TO PREVENT DRUG ABUSE BEFORE IT GROWS INTO A PROBLEM

Do you want to protect your child from drug abuse? It is important for parents to be aware of what causes drug abuse and how to stop it before it starts. Parents are going to be the first line of defense in this fight for their children.

According to the National Council on Alcoholism and Drug Dependence, "drug abuse is a term that refers to the use of illegal drugs or prescription medications for reasons other than those intended by the prescribing physician". This definition includes both legal and illegal drugs. However, among teenagers alcohol is involved in more drug abuse incidents than any other drug.

Parents should be aware of "normal" drug abuse so they can recognize any signs that their child is abusing drugs. The American Academy of Pediatrics, the Surgeon General's Report on Youth Violence and the National Institute on Drug Abuse all warn parents about the dangers of alcohol or other drugs among teenagers. When a parent sees a change in his child's behavior, he should talk to him about his changing behavior. If that doesn't work, he should seek professional help.

Parents must also recognize signs that the drug(s) being abused is illegal. The National Council on Alcoholism and Drug Dependence recommends that parents ask their children about drug use. It is surprising to learn that about 3 to 5 times as many teenagers who take illegal drugs admit to doing so in front of their parents than among those who do not.

Parents should be aware of the dangers of alcohol and other drugs among teenagers even though they may think their child is using them safely or "mindfully. It is also important to know what drugs are most likely to be used among teenagers and the problems they can cause.

To prevent drug abuse among teenagers, parents must get involved with their children's activities and hobbies. Parents should talk to their teenagers about activities that are important to them and support them in their choices.

Parents must also be aware of the possible dangers associated with illegal drug use by teenagers and understand the laws that govern the use of these drugs. This will allow you to give your child the proper guidance based on current laws.

Parents should educate themselves about drugs by reading books on the subject or watching educational videos on this subject. As parents learn about drugs, they can help their teenagers understand the dangers of drug use and show them that they are not alone in this fight for safe drug use.

THE NEED FOR MORE RESEARCH AND PROPER REGULATION OF DRUGS AGAINST THE BENEFITS THEY PROVIDE

The drugs we use to treat illnesses and diseases are being abused by people who want a high from them, often at the expense of their own health. The need for more research into the benefits and risks of these drugs is high now so that the trend of drug abuse can be curbed.

The need for research and proper regulation of drugs is a multi-dimensional issue. Drugs have several benefits, both medical and recreational. They are used for treating and curing diseases like diabetes, Parkinson's, Sclerosis etc. Modern pharmacology as a science has been able to treat several illnesses that were previously considered incurable by earlier methods of treatment. Drugs are also used to help people relax after a stressful day. These are just two of the many benefits provided by drugs.

The abuse of these drugs for recreation purposes is a dangerous trend that is on the rise in several countries around the world. People are using these drugs without knowledge of the side effects or proper dosage and in large quantities to get a high.

This leads to addiction and even death in several cases. The recreational use of drugs can also lead to psychological dependence.

Apart from the health related issues, there are several other dangers that come with recreational drug abuse. Law enforcement agencies have a tough time curbing drug smuggling and distribution leading to the proliferation of organized criminal networks. The social costs associated with these organizations are very high.

There is also a serious danger of the so-called designer drugs in this regard. These drugs are specially designed to bypass regulations with low dosages so as to make them legal and more easily available in the market. There is often a lack of proper knowledge about the usage and effects of these drugs.

Drug abuse also leads to financial costs that are borne by the public. These costs include those incurred by law enforcement agencies to curb drug trafficking and usage, and sometimes even the cost of treatment for addicts.

Legislation has been drafted by several countries against the use of drugs for recreational purposes by people without any medical need. However, these laws are often difficult to enforce and organized crime rings continue to manage their operations hoping to make large profits from these drugs.

The need for more research into the effects of drugs on the human body and their benefits is high. The benefits should be researched thoroughly so that they can be used to treat patients without jeopardizing their health. The side effects and long term effects of these drugs should also be studied.

The need for proper regulation of drugs is also very high. A multi-dimensional approach should be adopted so as to include quality control, production, distribution and regulation all at the same time. This will help in curbing drug use among the general population and also among the medical community.

One of the largest challenges in this regard is financial. Research into the benefits of drugs on human health is costly. The cost of researching all the possible drugs and their effects is high. Also, regulation in this context will be expensive. If the government chooses to completely outlaw recreational use of drugs, then large amounts of money will have to be spent for proper law enforcement and control over smuggling activities.

Research in this area should be a priority for all nations as people continue to abuse drugs for recreational purposes even though it impairs their physical and mental health.

THE ROLES OF PARENTS IN THE PREVENTION OF DRUG ABUSE AMONG CHILDREN AND ADOLESCENTS.

Parents are constantly warned about the harmful effects of drug abuse. Yet, most people don't realize that children can be introduced to drugs at a young age in the form of candy or medicine. They grow up with these drugs being used and abused around them and as a result, become addicts before they know what's happening. Parents need to be aware of what their children are doing and how to prevent drug abuse from occurring in the future.

"Talk to your kids about drugs and alcohol. Tell them what you are going to say ahead of time, and then stick to it. Keep the conversation short and age-appropriate. But don't forget that whatever age your child is, you need to keep the lines of communication open."

Although it may be embarrassing for a parent or adult friend to discuss drug use with young children, information about drug abuse can be valuable as they grow older. Children who grow up in a drug-free environment and attend school with high-achieving peers are less likely to experiment with drugs. They are also less likely to use drugs or alcohol if they are introduced by a friend who has already been drinking, smoking marijuana, or using cocaine. A child's attitude toward drugs depends on the other children in their social group who share similar attitudes.

"Focus on the fact that a drug-free household is best for everyone. Whatever you say, you will be remembered and the message will be passed down to your next-generation." There are many various methods that parents can keep their children from using drugs. One of the most important things they can do is to talk to their children about drugs and alcohol when they are young. This will allow them to learn about the risks involved with abuse and give them an opportunity to discuss it with a parent or person close to them as they grow older. Most parents won't be able to stop all drug abuse, but they will be able to make a difference with each child that grows up in a drug-free household.

"Drug-abuse is a problem that affects every family. It's never too late to start doing something about it."

There are many different types of drugs that can be abused. Whether it's prescription drugs, illegal drugs, or even alcohol, a child can be introduced to one of them at a young age. It is important for parents to learn about the different types of drug abuse so they can talk to their children about the dangers and educate them on how to stay away from them. Parents who want to stop the child from using drugs need to know how they work and what substances they contain in order for it to be effective. It is important for young children to recognize the different effects of certain drugs so they can avoid experimenting with them when they are older.

"Your involvement and unconditional love is what makes a difference in the life of your child, no matter who they are."

Teaching kids about drugs and alcohol is just as vital as teaching them how to drive safely or how to act appropriately in public. There are many different methods that parents can introduce their children to drug abuse. By learning about the different types of drugs and how they affect the human body, parents can prevent their children from ever using illegal substances before it's too late.

Children who grow up in a drug-free environment are less likely to experiment with drugs.

9

WHAT ARE THE POSSIBLE LEGAL CONSEQUENCES OF DRUG ABUSE?

According to the Supreme Court of the United States, drug abuse is any use of a drug in amounts that are not medically prescribed. Drug abuse may also be termed either Vicarious Liability for Drug-Involved Crimes or Negligent Infliction for Injury from Drug Use.

When you are under 18 years old, your parent or guardian should have full legal control over your life decisions. If they do not, they could be held legally liable and potentially imprisoned because of their child's drug abuse.

WHAT ARE THE LEGAL CONSEQUENCES FOR DRUG ABUSE OF ADOLESCENTS?

Under the newly passed Juvenile Justice and Delinquency Prevention Act, juvenile drug abuse will be punished more severely than in the past. The juvenile system is becoming increasingly punitive, including detention instead of probation. Punishments for juveniles may be as severe as 16 years imprisonment or even life imprisonment. Many states have adopted "Three Strikes and You're Out" laws that make it almost impossible to avoid prison time by pleading guilty to a drug-related crime.

WHAT ARE THE LEGAL CONSEQUENCES FOR ADULTS WHO ARE INVOLVED WITH DRUG ABUSE?

If you are already an adult, you will receive a harsher punishment than the juvenile counterpart. Many adult drug arrests can include jail time of at least one year or more. Also, you may have to serve this time and pay thousands of dollars in fines for the possession of drugs. You can receive a longer prison sentence if you sell or distribute these drugs, or if you are arrested with money and property related to drug trafficking.

Are there Different Kinds of Drug-Related Crimes?

For adults, there are three basic kinds of drug-related crime categories: possession, manufacture and sale.

If you plead guilty to possession, you may be sentenced to state prison for one year or more. If convicted of manufacture or sale, the term will generally range between 5 and 25 years. However, the penalties for manufacturing or selling will depend upon the type of drugs that you have manufactured or sold. For example, manufacturing crack cocaine may be punished more severely than manufacturing marijuana. You should check with an attorney to learn the exact penalties for these three felony crimes.

WHAT ARE THE LEGAL CONSEQUENCES IF I WAS INVOLVED IN A DRUG-RELATED ACCIDENT?

Although many people believe that it is legal to drive under the influence of drugs, this is not true. If you use drugs and drive, it is considered a crime. Consider this hypothetical example: if you are driving home from a party and another driver runs into your car because you were driving under the influence of drugs, then you could be held responsible for the other driver's injuries. It does not count whether or not that individual was actually injured, because your negligence caused them to be hurt. If there are no injuries, you may still be charged with endangerment.

The severity of the crime is determined by how many drugs were in your system and whether you could have been convicted of a felony offense if arrested. No matter how serious the offense, however, you will not receive a jail sentence unless you were under the influence of drugs at the time that the crime occurred.

WHAT ARE THE LEGAL CONSEQUENCES FOR MEDICAL MARIJUANA?

A marijuana-infused brownie or a joint can be just as illegal as one that contains crack cocaine. The penalties for possessing marijuana are based on its quantity and weight. The law specifies that it is anyone's right to grow, possess and use marijuana for personal use and medical purposes if allowed by a doctor's prescription. However, the law does not permit open-air public use. Many states such as Arizona, Washington and Oregon have passed laws that allow the personal consumption of small amounts of marijuana in the privacy of their own homes, but still prevent people from consuming it outdoors.

WHAT ARE THE LEGAL CONSEQUENCES FOR NON-MEDICAL USE OF PRESCRIPTION DRUGS?

Prescription drugs have become a multi-billion industry. Almost every kind of drug used to treat pain, depression or anxiety is available from pharmacies and on the internet without doctor's orders. The legal ramifications of this misuse are great. If you are arrested for using prescription drugs without a prescription, you may be charged with either a misdemeanor or felony depending on the state laws. Generally, if the amount of drugs is less than 10 grams, then it is considered a misdemeanor and you are likely to receive less harsh penalties.

Additional consequences may include probation or home confinement, heavy fines and community service.

THE DIFFERENT TYPES OF PENALTIES FOR DRUG OFFENSES

In the United States, penalties for drug offenses are determined by how severe the offense is. The penalty depends on whether it's a felony or a misdemeanor. Felony penalties include fines, lengthy jail sentences, prison sentences of one year or more, and life imprisonment. The possible maximum term of imprisonment for a misdemeanor conviction is less than one year and does not include any potential imprisonment in state prison.

Drug offenses are categorized into two different classes. The two classes are status offenses and violent crimes. As a status offense, the penalties for drug offenses include fines, community service, probation and/or parole. Violent crimes include felonies such as assault or murder that involve drugs; they also include other drug-related crimes such as prostitution and possession of narcotics with intent to distribute them.

The amount of the fine greatly changes depending on the type of drug offence. The minimum fine for an offense involving a controlled substance is $1,000. For a felony of the first degree, the minimum fine is $2,000; for felonies of the second and third degrees, fines range from $1,000 to $25,000. The highest penalty for possession with the intent to distribute a controlled substance is life imprisonment and a fine of at least $100,000. The penalty for possession of cocaine or heroin with intent to distribute them is also life imprisonment and a fine of at least $100,000.

The law specifies the maximum amount of fines that a person can be convicted of under state and federal law. The maximum possible fine for drug offenses in federal court is $1,000,000.

The consequences for a conviction on misdemeanor drug charges include imprisonment of less than one year and a fine of less than $2,500. The possible penalty for a felony offense is not prison time but could include imprisonment up to 10 years or more or fines up to $10,000. If the conviction is for a violent crime such as murder or rape, the penalty will depend on the severity of the crime.

Under U.S. federal law, it is also possible to have a person's professional license suspended or revoked if they are convicted of drug abuse, this can occur in any of three different ways:

In almost all states, it is considered illegal to drive while under the influence of alcohol or other drugs. A few states allow the offense to be referred to as "driving under the influence" (DUI), "driving while intoxicated" (DWI) or "operating while intoxicated" (OWI). The penalties for this offense vary from state to state.

The penalties given for driving under the influence vary greatly from state to state. It is also possible for a driver's vehicle to be impounded (usually for 30 days in most states). Penalties can include fines and the suspension or revocation of a person's driver's license. Drivers may also be ordered to attend alcohol or drug counseling (often referred to as "DUI School" in some states).

Drug Trafficking Penalties

The penalties for drug trafficking are severe because traffickers can potentially make millions of dollars selling illicit drugs. In some states, the penalty for drug trafficking is a prison sentence which may exceed 20 years. The minimum penalty for trafficking of cocaine or heroin is at least 10 years in prison.

In the United States, drug traffickers are considered to be one of the most serious criminals and may be subjected to longer prison sentences than other criminals. Many drug traffickers are put in maximum-security prisons, isolated from the general prison population. It is also common for drug traffickers to be placed in solitary confinement because they are seen as a threat to security in most prisons.

For example, in Florida, possession of more than 25 grams of cocaine (or any amount of narcotics) automatically constitutes trafficking. In Indiana, trafficking in illegal narcotics is a Class B felony which carries a minimum sentence of 10 years in prison if the amount of narcotics involved is 28 grams or more.

Laws against drug trafficking and abuse are generally very strict in the United States, and people convicted of drug offenses are subjected to mandatory minimum sentencing laws. The federal government also imposes harsh penalties for drug-related offenses. For example, individuals convicted of distributing one gram or more of heroin receive a mandatory minimum sentence of five years in prison under federal law.

In many states, persons caught transporting drugs face harsher penalties than those who use or sell drugs themselves. This is because the drug trafficking penalties are reserved for large drug cartels and other large-scale distribution operations.

In some states, the penalties are so severe that drug dealers are sometimes punished with life imprisonment. This is true in several states, including Florida, Georgia, Louisiana, New Hampshire and Texas.

In addition to drug trafficking and other drug-related crimes, drug offenses also may be associated with weapons possession or sale or a violent act. The penalties for these crimes vary greatly from state to state; however, the most severe penalties usually are reserved for dealers of large quantities of illegal drugs such as cocaine or heroin. Offenders who are convicted of dealing in large quantities can face sentences of many years in prison.

HOW LONG DO CONVICTED DRUG ABUSERS SPEND IN JAIL?

There are many different factors to consider when discussing the length of a prison sentence. In America, the legality of drugs also plays a large part in determining how long someone will serve behind bars for drug-related crimes.

What crimes qualify as drug-related, how long convicted drug abusers spend in jail and finally some words about whether or not they have a chance at rehabilitation. I will start by discussing the severity of drug-related crimes and then the length of sentences associated with them.

When deciding on a prison sentence for a drug related crime, one must take into consideration all three of these factors:

1. Was the defendant legally intoxicated at the time?
   Depending on what type of drugs were involved, this will influence the outcome.
2. How much and what type of drugs were involved? The more severe the drug abuse, the longer the sentence is likely to be.
3. The defendant's age and past history. An older drug abuser is much more likely to have a greater

punishment then a younger one who had a similar life-experience.

What qualifies as a drug related crime?

There are different offenses considered "drug related" in the court system. These include crimes that involved, were used in the process of, or were discovered by a law enforcement officer as a result of a drug related investigation.

The majority of drug related crimes are serious offenses that involve hard drugs such as: cocaine, heroin or methamphetamine. These crimes include possession with intent to distribute (PID) and trafficking. However, there are less severe drug related crimes such as dealing prescription drugs like OxyContin for example (a painkiller).

A person who is convicted of a drug related offense will likely serve time in prison. However, the amount of time they spend behind bars depends on the severity of the crime. A person who was convicted of a misdemeanor involving drugs will likely spend no more than one year in prison. When individuals are convicted of a felony drug charge, they will possibly spend from two to five years in jail.

You may also be required to serve time in a rehab program such as Narcotics Anonymous (NA) or attend Alcoholics Anonymous (AA) in order to qualify for parole. This is usually the case if your drug problems were considered a main reason for your criminal activity. The length of an AA/NA meeting is usually around one hour.

A person who has been convicted of a drug related crime will likely serve time in prison, but the length of their stay depends on the severity of their offense.

How long a person spends in prison can also depend on the type of drugs they were accused of dealing. For example, if a person is convicted of dealing prescription drugs they may be sent to a rehab center instead of having to serve time in prison.

If someone is convicted of trafficking hard drugs like cocaine or heroin, there is a possibility that they could be sentenced to life in prison without parole. This means that the judge will lock them up for the rest of their natural lives.

How Long Do Drug Abusers Spend in Jail?

If you are busted for drug possession, the number of months you spend in prison depends on the drug type, weight and your record. For example, a person who is caught with marijuana will likely spend two to six months in prison. A person found with cocaine could be looking at an additional eight to sixteen months in jail.

If you are convicted of trafficking hard drugs (cocaine, opiates, meth or heroin) you will likely be sentenced to a minimum of 10 years before a parole board decides if you qualify for release.

You may also find yourself being sentenced to life without parole.

Drug Possession Penalties (Length of Sentence)

As previously mentioned, the penalties for drug possession depend upon the type of drug involved. The lighter the substance, the less severe your sentence is likely to be. Common drugs that carry serious sentences include: methamphetamine, heroin and cocaine.

The length of your sentence may also depend on your past crimes and the charges presented against you and your criminal record. For example, if you have a history of drug possession, you will likely serve longer then someone who does not have a criminal history.

The severity of your drug crime may also affect your sentence. For example, if you are sentenced to a life sentence without parole you will have to spend the rest of your life in prison.

Is Drug Treatment an Option?

While some people believe that drug treatment is not an option, there are many programs available throughout the United States. A person who received a clean record for drug abuse treatment may not be put behind bars if they come across as a good candidate for rehabilitation.

In the case of possession crimes, a treatment center may be able to offer drug or alcohol rehabilitation as an alternative to prison. This is a realistic option and it may make sense to go this route, even if there are other circumstances that make you ineligible for treatment (like lack of health insurance).

For example, if your past is littered with alcohol and drug related issues, but you have decided to enter treatment, the judge may not sentence you to prison. This is because the judge realizes that you had a problem and you were able to get over it.

Drug Treatment Programs

Drug treatment programs are a great option for people who are facing drug or alcohol related charges in court. These programs will give you an opportunity to get the help that you need in order to stay sober, without having to spend time behind bars. Nevertheless, it is very essential to remember that if the program fails, you could be facing more prison time than before.

If you or a loved one is facing charges related to drug possession, it is important to know your options. It is also important to know the charges that you are facing and how this may affect your sentencing. Once you have been accused of a crime, you are entitled to speak with a criminal defense lawyer. The attorney can help assess the severity of your situation and guide you towards the best possible outcome.

REHABILITATION PROGRAMS WITHIN THE JAIL SYSTEM

There is a common misconception that jail is the only place where drug abusers go to receive treatment. However, rehabilitation programs within the jail system have helped significantly reduce drug abuse, crime and recidivism. With programs like these, inmates are provided with incentives to engage in different activities such as drug testing and counseling which can help them look forward to a successful future.

The common misconception that jail is the only place where drug addicts go for rehabilitation has been proven false by the existence of programs within jails. There are three main portions of the drug program within a jail: order, structure and incentives. The order involves the drugs being brought into a controlled environment to prevent them being smuggled in from the outside. Then, there must be a structured timetable for the inmates to follow over their two-year stay within which they should have at least six classes every week. Finally, there are incentives for the inmates to engage in activities that will provide them with personal gains. If they maintain a healthy lifestyle and have a good record, they could be rewarded with telephone privileges, an allowance or even being moved to a less-secure facility.

These rehabilitation programs within the jail system can reduce violence and substance abuse in the inmate population because it allows them to focus on their mental health. For these programs to be implemented in jails, the jails must be able to provide facilities for the inmates to take part in. More often than not, these facilities should include recreational activities such as video games and sports; however, they could also be provided with psychological treatment.

Once a prisoner is released into society after serving their jail terms, there are many ways in which they can receive treatment. One of the first steps that they need to take is by completing a drug assessment form that will help them identify their drug of choice and the dosage. Once this is done, it will help them to take a more active role in the treatment process. The next step that they need to take is to enroll in an emergency pilot program which will give them the opportunity to meet with a specialist who can provide them with guidance on staying fit and healthy. Finally, there are numerous places that they can go for further assistance which deals with treatment options for their specific drug of choice.

There have been many rehab programs within jails in order to combat drug abuse. One of the most effective programs is the Drug Distribution Program (DDP) which has been proven to reduce drug abuse within inmates. This program allows for those who are in jail to receive their medication from the jails and not from their homes where they could have a higher risk of abusing them. It has also benefited inmates because they are less likely to share their medication with someone else if they had received it from the jail.

For those who do leave jail with an addiction that requires medical attention, there are many different treatment options available. One of the most common options is a relapse prevention program which involves medication and counseling. The medications that are used are not addictive and will lead to an overall better mental health for the patient—this means that there is less chance of them relapse. Another option that can be used is the Methadone Maintenance Therapy (MMT) which relies on a combination of medication and counseling in order to help patients overcome their addiction. It also can be used to help patients maintain their life outside of jail and keep them from relapsing when they leave jail.

Those people who are addicted to prescription drugs can come into contact with a medication case manager which will help them to find the best treatment program for their medical condition. The case manager will help them to receive prescriptions for their medication from the pharmacy and assist them with completing any forms that they need. This can also be used if they don't have a prescription but want to obtain one. Some of the medications that these case managers can help with include Xanax and Ativan. For those who need treatment for their addiction to prescription drugs, there are many different options available to them through their medication case manager.

The Bureau of Justice Assistance has made a program that can help inmates find employment after they leave jail. This program is called the Faith-Based Re-Entry Employment Services (FRES) which allows for inmates to find work with a faith-based organization such as churches or any other religious based organizations. It is important that the inmates find jobs that they can work at after they leave jail because it will increase their chances of avoiding a relapse as well as reducing their chances of returning to jail. The funds provided through this program go towards the inmates and finding them job leads.

Another program intended to help inmates find employment is the Department of Labor's Reentry Employment Services (RES) which allows for them to search for a wide variety of jobs, including those that are not faith based. It can also help inmates who are looking for general assistance in finding work, such as resume building, or training. The Department of Labor will assist inmates in finding a job by providing them with a wide variety of job leads that they can use to search for employment.

For those who are released from jail without an addiction but still use drugs or alcohol, the best way to avoid relapsing is to find a sober living facility. These facilities provide a place for the recovering addict to go that can prevent them from relapsing, while also providing them with the resources that they need to stay sober. These facilities also provide therapy for those who live in them and can be used after they have transitioned back into society.

The resources included in sober living facilities vary by facility. Some places provide help with the rehab process such as outpatient drug treatment. Others provide programs, such as the one that has been successful in prison and jail settings called Aftercare, which can help the recovering addict stay sober after leaving jail. Many of these facilities offer therapy for the recovering addict and also job training to help them find work when they are ready to transition back into society.

WHAT IS THE COST OF DRUG ABUSE TO SOCIETY?

Drug abuse is linked to crime, violence, mental health issues, and a variety of medical conditions. The National Institute on Drug Abuse estimates that the societal cost of drug abuse in the United States is more than 1 trillion dollars.

There are many unintended social consequences associated with drug abuse that can affect people on an individual level as well as society as a whole. Drug abuse can affect employment, income, and personal relationships.

Drug abuse is not only a problem with the individual who is abusing drugs, but also with his or her family members and co-workers. The NIDA estimates that drug use alone costs society $193 billion per year. This does not include medical costs or lost productivity due to addiction. The NIDA's estimate is based on a cost-of-illness approach, which takes into account medical treatment and lost income due to unemployment or underemployment. The NIDA also breaks down the cost of drug abuse among people ages 12 and older into individual categories. The most expensive costs associated with drug use are those associated with criminal justice, such as police and prisons, as well as lost productivity at work.

The NIDA estimates a loss of income among people ages 12 and older who report drug abuse. The NIDA notes the highest unemployment rate of those with drug abuse issues is 22 percent. Approximately 90 percent of those who gain employment eventually lose it, either because of loss of a job due to substance abuse or because they voluntarily quit their job to avoid work related conflicts caused by substance abuse.

NIDA also shows the great costs associated with employment in those who use illegal drugs. The NIDA estimates that employers lose $65.8 billion each year due to employees who use illegal drugs. This number is based on income lost due to productivity and unemployment or underemployment, as well as the cost of healthcare associated with drug abuse.

The NIDA estimates that $56 billion in healthcare costs are incurred by people of all ages who abuse drugs. Each year over one million people abuse prescription medications, which account for $28.5 billion in healthcare costs associated with drug abuse issues. An additional $16.9 billion in healthcare costs are incurred because of dependence on alcohol.

The NIDA estimates that criminal justice costs for drug abuse reach $8.5 billion a year. This number is based on police intervention and prosecution, as well as the cost of prisons, probation, and parole for those involved with drug abuse issues.

Individuals who use illegal drugs or misuse prescription medications have an increased risk of contracting a wide range of diseases and disorders. Drug abuse increases the risk of contracting infectious diseases such as HIV/ AIDS, Hepatitis C, and syphilis. Drug use is also linked to a wide range of mental health issues, such as mood disorders and schizophrenia.

Drug abuse is also associated with a number of medical conditions that usually require costly medical treatment, such as chronic health conditions. The NIDA reports that 20 percent of all hospital stays are for drug-related issues. Individuals who use illegal drugs may also require treatment for injuries sustained from accidents caused by their drug abuse.

The NIDA estimates that the direct economic loss for drug abuse in the United States was $193 billion a year. The NIDA breaks down these costs among those ages 12 and older into categories, including criminal justice, healthcare, and quality of life (employment).

The National Institute on Drug Abuse accounts that there are many indirect costs associated with drug abuse that are difficult to measure. For example, substance abuse can cause people to skip school or work, which decreases their income. Substance abuse can also increase the likelihood that a family member will be incarcerated, which leads to loss of income.

The NIDA notes that some of the indirect costs for drug abuse are not quantifiable. Social costs associated with drug use include crime and violence, health and mental health issues, as well as relationship problems between co-workers and employers who have an employee who is abusing drugs.

THE COSTS OF DRUG ABUSE IN MEDICAL-RELATED EXPENDITURE

According to the DEA's "The Economic Impact of Drug Control Spending in the United States", there was a total of $28.5 billion dollars spent on medical-related expenditure. Medical related expense is defined as any health care expenditures that are directly linked to drug abuse. This can include hospital costs, doctor visits, outpatient treatment, and prescription medication as a result of drug abuse.

This number does not include the costs of law enforcement or incarceration related to drug abuse.

The costs of drug abuse are very high and contribute to a great deal of financial difficulty in the United States. Medical-related expenditure for drug related illness is estimated to be $13 billion dollars. This number shows that the majority of medical-related expenditure in relation to drug abuse is spent on substance abuse treatment. The majority (63 percent) of all medical-related expenditure was spent on drug treatment through health care services and mental health services most specifically. Another 23 percent of all medical-related expenditure was spent on testing, education, and prevention. The amount of medical-related expenditure closely correlates with society's belief that drug abuse is a serious disease that must be treated as such and treated accordingly. The presumption that drug abuse is a disease that needs to be understood and treated is not necessarily true but the situation can be defused by addressing the problem at hand. In order to prevent further financial issues, society needs to improve public awareness of the costs of drug abuse and the benefits it inflicts on society.

The statistics can be very revealing when they are analyzed. The cost for a drug abuser over his/her lifetime varies depending upon the type of drug used, how often it is consumed, and how often there is a variety of drugs used. The percentage of time spent being sick is also very significant in these numbers. The average cost of a drug abuser is between $35,000 and $50,000 for every year he/she is abusing drugs. The number varies from a low of $1,000 per year if the drug abuser only uses marijuana to an average of $3,500 per year for cocaine abuse. If there are no health related expenses then the total average cost is around $33,750.

The medical costs associated with drug abuse are very high and very costly to society in general. However, the medical costs are very misleading because they do not consider the fact that many people can be "addicted" to prescription drugs. In some cases of addiction, there may not be a significant financial cost involved for the individual, but there is still an effect on personal life and family expenses. Though it would appear as though people using these prescription drugs were more likely to abuse them or even become addicted, it does not explain why they must use them in order for them to function normally or at all. It is vital that people understand the potential of prescription drugs and not assume that they can never be abused, but understand that for every one person abusing any drug there are a vast amount who are abusing prescription drugs.

Some of the costs that might be associated with drug abuse include the itemized medical expenses in which people end up incurring from using illegal drugs and prescription drugs. These costs can include the cost of drug related illnesses, treatment in general, and the decreased quality of life when using illicit drugs. People do not need to be continually using illegal drugs in order for them to suffer from a drug-related illness. These costs are very real and very detrimental.

One of the costs that are very devastating to individuals who have used illicit drugs is a condition known as a drug overdose. Drug overdoses are the leading cause of non-fatal injuries in the United States and can be fatal. The number of deaths caused by drug overdoses has been on a dramatic rise over the past few years. Approximately, 60,000 Americans die from drug overdoses every year. Overdose deaths are not limited to illegal drugs; overdose can also be caused by prescription drugs. Drug overdose does not just affect the individual using illicit drugs or prescription drugs but also has an effect on the surrounding people and society in general.

These numbers do not reflect all of the actual costs that are related to drug abuse since only certain types of cost are included in these statistics.

Another important cost that is associated with illicit drugs is a disease known as HIV/AIDS. Illicit drug use puts users at a high risk of contracting the disease. The number one cause of this condition is sharing contaminated needles. This puts drug abusers in a much more dangerous situation since it can lead to life-threatening diseases such as AIDS. It is very important for individuals to follow the rules concerning needle use and other drugs in order to prevent HIV/AIDS. Co-infection can occur during intravenous drug use and other intravenous drug-related procedures. This can be prevented by using clean needles and by not sharing needles that are used for intravenous drug use.

Another cost to society that is not necessarily reflected in these statistics is the lost potential of many individuals who use drugs. Illicit drug use prevents people from being able to reach their full potentials because of the negative effects it has on their lives. This also makes it more difficult for many individuals to obtain jobs or even attend school. The increased costs associated with illicit drug use prevent individuals from being able to pursue their goals and dreams. People may lose out on these opportunities because they have chosen to use illicit drugs.

THE EFFECTS OF DRUG ABUSE ON PROFESSIONAL PERFORMANCE

Drug abuse could negatively affect the professional success of an athlete, as well as his or her personal life. The effects of drug and alcohol consumption can seem very difficult to cure, especially if it is prevalent in people's lives. Drug use will leave the person feeling numb and out of touch with reality, which could lead to dangerous behaviors such as reckless driving or other criminal acts. These risks may cause a loss in their potential career earnings because they are not performing well on the field causing them to lose opportunities for endorsements. Not only that, an athlete could also face legal problems such as driving under the influence (DUI) and possibly being arrested.

If a player chooses to use drugs or alcohol, it could affect his or her performance on the field. An athlete who is using drugs may not be able to control his or her emotions while the person is playing, which can lead to making mistakes that can cost the team valuable points in a game. The player may not be able to think quickly or strategize like he or she could while sober. If a player is on drugs, then they are more likely to commit errors due to the fact that their heart rate could be elevated, making them unable to think as clearly and react as fast as they normally would without the use of drugs or alcohol.

Drugs and alcohol can also cause mood swings in the player, causing them to become aggressive and irrational. Typically, all athletes have some level of anger issues. When an athlete is angry, they may not be able to control their emotions, which could get them kicked out of a game and result in a suspension. If the player has a volatile temper, then he or she could be suspended by the league or put into early retirement. This anger issue can also be a source of stress for the athlete off the field dealing with family and friends who may be uncomfortable around him or her due to their unstable behaviors that spiral out of control.

Experiencing an addiction to a drug or alcohol is also very stressful for the person using. The person may experience anxiety if they don't have access to the drug or they will feel sick if they try to stop using. The side effects can be detrimental and hurt an athlete's performance and their personal lives as well.

If you are abusing drugs and alcohol at work, it is likely that you have a higher chance of getting injured, or worse getting fired. Which means that your company will lose out on money. It's not just about the cost of replacing a worker though; drug abuse also has a corrosive effect on productivity. Drug and alcohol abuse often has people make mistakes in their work that cost money.

Lost productivity in the workplace due to drug abuse is a significant issue. The Center for Substance Abuse Research states that substance abuse cost each year is $166 billion out of the $1.4 trillion that U.S. employers pay their employees annually (Costs).

One area that falls under the suppresses effects of drug abuse is performance. Drug abuse can cause people to behave in ways that will keep them from performing their job effectively; sometimes it causes them to lose their job. All too often employers find that drug users are disruptive, and they often have little respect for authority. Employees with addictions may be unable or unwilling to stay on task or focused during the working day. As a result, employers simply cannot trust them with the important responsibilities of their job, which is why they are ultimately laid off.

The unfortunate part of drug abuse is that the consequences can negatively impact people's careers in a lot of different ways. Some of the common negative effects include:

- Loss of productivity
- Loss of profits in the form of profits due to mismanagement or breakdown in operations
- Reduced motivation and motivation loss due to lack of attention or focus
- Possible job termination for an employee because they are unable to meet a particular standard, and

performance is negatively affected by drugs and alcohol
use.

- Legal problems which are resulting from drug or
  alcohol use on the job.
- Increased likelihood of accidents that result in injuries
  or death.

To avoid the negative effects of drug and alcohol abuse on
career, it's important to seek help before it affects your life.

11

HOW CAN WE DETERMINE THE IMPACT OF DRUG ABUSE ON SOCIETY?

Drug abuse is a very serious problem that affects both the individual and society as a whole. In accordance with the National Institute on Drug Abuse, drug abuse is an expensive public health issue and causes serious damage to both individuals and society. Drug addiction has negative effects on one's physical health, mental health, employment status, marital status, financial security, school success in children of parents with addiction issues.

The human impact of drug abuse is enormous and often overlooked. The physical and mental problems resulting from drug abuse are not only devastating but irreparable as well.

Drug abuse and addiction are not problems that only the individual needs to deal with. They create hardship for their families and society as a whole.

Many individuals who have struggled with alcohol or drug addiction have difficulty finding a job, keeping a job, and staying sober once they do find a job. Strained relationships, lost homes, failed businesses, accidents and crimes are all results of drug abuse. The health care cost of treating individuals with drug addiction issues is significant; this cost is shared by all American citizens via tax dollars. The impact that drug abuse has on society is significant and systemic.

Imagine if every constituent in the United States could read about these statistics, then incorporate them into their daily lives. Imagine if they realized how their lives are directly impacted by the human toll that drugs and alcohol wreak upon others.

With all of this knowledge, it is no wonder drug abuse is still a widespread issue in the United States. It is important that all Americans recognize and attempt to reduce the prevalence of drug abuse. If we can stop drug abuse before it has begun, the cost to both society and individuals will be less than if we wait until it has already reached critical proportions.

The life span of an addict ranges from 3-9 years, depending on the severity and type of addiction. When you compare this to the life span of a non-addict, which is about 70 years, drug addiction is a quick ticket to death. Drug use leads to death and disease in many ways. It causes cancers, heart disease, and respiratory diseases.

There are many effects that abuse has on society, but the most devastating are the broken families and children. People who use drugs are more likely to have children that are neglected or abused.

Drugs kill innocent people everyday in ways that we cannot even begin to imagine. Drug use is not only very dangerous to the abuser, but it also makes them very dangerous to others. It is not uncommon for drug addicts to lose all control of their situations, which can lead them to take advantage of others in very harmful ways. A drug addict is not able to care for himself, much less others.

The human impact of drug abuse cannot be overstated. The reality is that drug addiction is a complicated problem that the individual, society, and families all need to address. What other problems do we wish to not solve but by ignoring them?

The U.S. Surgeon General has made a statement regarding drug use in America, saying that "drug use has a very serious impact on American society..." This is an important statement because it brings to light the consequences of drug use on our lives and our loved ones.

A drug addict has the potential of creating life-long problems in the lives of others. It is important that we all work together to reduce the damage that a drug addict can do to us.

The legacy of a drug addict is one that will continue to affect society until another generation is born and old enough to cope with the problems of their parents. We will all pay for the mistakes of drug addicts with our taxes. This is a cost that we would all love to avoid.

We can overcome the problem of drug addiction by informing ourselves and each other about the consequences of drug addiction.

This is an issue that should be of the highest priority for all Americans. Each one of us needs to make an effort to reduce drug abuse in our nation. It is not an issue that one group or government agency will be able to solve. We need to work together as a society and as individuals in order for this problem to be solved quickly and fairly.

When we all work together to solve this problem, we will be able to save money, improve the quality of our lives and our families' lives, and improve our society.

Drugs have a complex impact on society. It wakes up the community, puts people in harm's way and threatens the well-being of society by putting all citizens at risk of a host of diseases due to the toxins in drugs. However, the community can do a lot to stop drug-related crimes. They can help fight the effects of addiction by recognizing that drug users are being made sick by their own actions and they need help.

The United States is known as a "free" society, but there are many forms of exploitation that go on in our country. These exploitations include sex slavery and pornography, and perhaps the most difficult widespread problem to realize is that of drug addiction.

Drugs are a problem in the United States. There is no question about that. But just because there are so many drug addicts in our country doesn't mean that we can't do anything about it to change the statistics and help these individuals. If we don't stand up and fight for our rights, a lot of these addicts will never get better, and we'll always have to live with the consequences.

An addict will never stop taking drugs until he truly desires to do so. We all have to realize that drug addiction is a disease and not a crime. It is a sickness, like cancer or diabetes, where if the body is strong enough it can fight off the disease. People suffering from this disease need our understanding and support. They need our compassion and our love because they're not bad people: they're sick people.

We don't have very much control over what's going on in the world today. We all need to do what we can do to change the future. If we don't stand up for our rights, no one will.

I have seen many people die from drug addiction because they did not have a way of getting help. I am always trying to get the word out in my school that everyone should know what is going on in this world. We are not taught about reality, but we are always being led into it by the entertainment industry and other forms of propaganda that we are exposed to.

This is a problem that will not be solved in a day, or even a week for that matter. It may take years to solve but with the help of our community, we can get over this hump and prevent other families from going through what our family has gone through.

12

WHAT IS THE OUTLOOK FOR THE FUTURE IN REGARDS TO PREVENTING AND TREATING DRUG ABUSE?

In today's world, drug abuse is a prevalent issue which affects many people of all ages. Prevention and treatment programs are needed to help lessen the impacts that drugs have on society. We will explore the perspective in regards to preventing and treating drug abuse in order to limit the negative impact it has on society.

The more information individuals have about how drug addiction works, the less likely they are to think they can use drugs once or twice without becoming addicted themselves.

Drugs such as illegal drugs have been around for a long time and many people are afraid to question why the majority of people who abuse drugs do not use more socially accepted substances such as alcohol. The primary reason that many people think they will use drugs after using them once or twice is because they use them in a way that is not physically harmful or harmful emotionally. In this way, drug abusers often think they will be able to stop when the effects of the drug wear off. One of the biggest issues surrounding drug abuse is the frequency of drug use. If a person uses drugs, they will become physically dependent or psychologically dependent on them. This leads to addiction and once a person is addicted to drugs, they will not be able to stop using them without outside help and support. The more information that is given to the public about the effects of drugs, the more likely they are to understand what they are putting into their bodies and why it can cause them to become addicted. If they do not have this information, and they give in to peer pressure, then they may not be aware of what other effects drug abuse can have on a person's life.

The outlook for the future in regards to preventing and treating drug abuse is that it will improve. With doctors and researchers understanding the brain much better than they had in the past, medical treatments for addiction are more effective. Dual diagnosis treatment centers are also being used to treat both physical and mental health conditions, such as depression or anxiety that often co-occur with addiction.

A new treatment approach is pharmacological extinction, which is an important basic-science discovery that has the potential to revolutionize addiction treatment. As opposed to focusing on the addictive behavior, this approach targets the actual drug addiction, using medications that interfere with drug craving and relapse. Pharmacological extinction involves giving addicted patients a drug, such as a blocker of opioid or dopamine receptors, during relapse prevention therapy. This treatment interferes with the pleasure normally associated with an addictive substance, so that users learn to prefer less pleasurable non-drug options. This treatment now holds great promise for treating addiction.

In regards to treatment, more individuals are finding that going through outpatient programs work better for their recovery than admission in inpatient facilities. Those who go through outpatient programs tend to have fewer problems with substance abuse compared to those who are admitted into inpatient programs. It's really essential to find the right treatment program that will work for you.

Many people are still trying to find an effective treatment program for drug addiction, which is why it is important that you get the right one. Find one that you are comfortable with, and stick to the treatment plan. No matter what program you go through, seek professional help from a trained counselor or therapist to get the most out of it.

Drug abuse is a medical problem that can be treated in a variety of ways. Drug abuse prevention and education should begin at home, on the playground or in school; they should also be continued throughout adulthood through educational programs and public awareness strategies. With the correct education and treatment, parents and family members may be able to help their friends and family members recover from drug addiction. Drug addiction can be treated with a combination of therapy, rehabilitation, counseling, medication, group therapy or medication-assisted therapy. There are three main types of drug abuse treatment: inpatient, outpatient and residential. Inpatient treatment offers patients a structured environment where they can completely focus on their recovery. The level of care patients receive in an inpatient facility ranges from low intensity to therapeutic community or locked-down, depending on the patient's needs. Outpatient treatment is appropriate for those who can manage their addiction without professional help on a full-time basis. Outpatient treatment programs have the least amount of controls, and have less supervision and discipline compared to a residential treatment program. Residential treatment places patients in a center or house outside of their home, where they live with other addicts recovering together. This gives patients the best at-home experience possible.

Treatment centers are known for their individualized treatment plans and therapy techniques. Drug abuse treatment programs vary by the severity of addiction, type and age of patient as well as location choice. While inpatient programs can be expensive, outpatient programs offer some financial assistance and can be found throughout the U.S.

If you assume that you or a loved one has a drug problem, do not wait any longer to seek the help that you need. If you don't know where to turn, contact your doctor today and ask for a referral to a drug abuse treatment program. Ultimately, your decision to get help and begin recovery is one of the most important steps in defeating drug addiction.

Your family physician can offer valuable advice about treatment options for addiction and can recommend qualified professionals who are trained in these treatment programs.

Drug abuse is a global epidemic that requires a global response. Governments and international organizations should work together to establish a strong global framework that will support drug abuse prevention, treatment and rehabilitation. Additionally, they should target policies toward prevention and treatment needs, recognize the importance of family and community involvement, the need to develop international partnerships and work together to address the problem.

The challenge is to better understand drug addiction. It is also important to understand how drug addiction affects both individual lives and the health community as a whole. The medical community needs to come together in order for a global strategy for combating drug abuse to be effective. There needs to have a comprehensive plan in place that will prevent and treat drug addiction.

With a better understanding of drug addiction, and how it affects lives, the medical community will hopefully continue to improve treatment plans and find better ways to combat this disease. A global strategy will be necessary to effectively fight future drug abuse epidemics. In order to prevent and treat drug abuse, it is essential that the medical community work together and continue to make progress in individualized care for those with substance abuse issues. It is also important to spread awareness about substance abuse treatment and prevention methods. If we come together as a global community of professionals, we can make a difference in the lives of our patients.

CONCLUSION

Drug abuse may have a devastating effect on those involved with the drug as well as society in general. Drug abuse can lead to addiction, which is characterized by its ability to take over one's life and interfere with his or her social functioning. Addiction is not a rare disease. Out of every seven or eight individuals in American, there are at least one person with an addiction. In fact, it has been estimated that addiction affects one in five people that are attending treatment centers for drug abuse.

Drug abuse can lead to addiction, which in turn leads to a higher risk of mortality. Death from drug overdose, death by violence and an increased susceptibility of other diseases is also associated with the effects of drug abuse. Just looking at these statistics, it is very easy to see how abuse can affect the quality of life for those afflicted with addiction and can also have a negative effect on society. However, addiction does not only affect those who use drugs. It is also associated with loss of productivity and poor decision making that can lead to other negative consequences.

When a person becomes addicted to drugs, his or her family may experience psychological and financial problems. Addiction can also affect a person's career and social life, which will eventually result in poor decision making. Ultimately, the poor decisions made by drug addicts often lead to their arrest through illegal activity done in order to support their addiction. Their arrest can leave them with legal problems that will further affect their lives and eventually, if an addict continues to use illegal substances, he or she can end up incarcerated which further affects his or her future.

There are many problems that occur as a result of the use of drugs that are not readily visible. The psychological effects of drugs can be devastating as well to an individual's psyche and can lead to the deterioration of a person's entire life. Even with the negative consequences of drug abuse, though, it is still an extremely difficult habit to break. It is estimated that only 10% of all people who enter treatment centers for drug abuse ever get clean and sober. Therefore, it is vitally important that more people are made aware of the harmful effects of drugs and this book is not only motivate those who think about taking drugs to quit their use, but it also prompt those who use drugs to seek help.

Although drug abuse does not have many visible consequences, however it can still have a devastating effect on those dealing with the addiction and those around them. The social and economic effects can be just as harmful as the psychological issues faced by those with drug abuse problems. More people need to become aware of the devastating effects that result from drug use and in order for this awareness to be effective action needs to be taken. Drug abuse is hard to stop without the help of others but the dangers are worth the risk. So if you or someone you know is dealing with drug addiction it is important to get help as soon as possible.

It is not easy to quit taking drugs, but it can be done with the proper amount of determination and the right resources. With a combination of the proper attitude and assistance, drug addiction can be conquered and those who have been affected by drugs can lead a normal life.

GLOSSARY

Ambenonium (as ambenonium dichloride, trade name Mytelase) is a cholinesterase inhibitor used in the management of myasthenia gravis.

Atropine is a tropane alkaloid and anticholinergic medication used to treat certain types of nerve agent and pesticide poisonings as well as some types

Benadryl is a brand of various antihistamine medications used to stop allergies, whose content varies in different countries, but which includes some or no combination of diphenhydramine, acrivastine, and cetirizine.

Benzodiazepines (BZD, BDZ, BZs), sometimes called "benzos", are a class of psychoactive drugs whose core chemical structure is the fusion of a benzene ring and a diazepine ring. As depressants—drugs which lower brain activity—they are prescribed to treat conditions such as anxiety, insomnia, seizures.

Bioavailability (BA or F) is a subcategory of absorption and is the fraction (%) of an administered drug that reaches the systemic circulation.

Buprenorphine is an opioid used to treat opioid use disorder, acute pain, and chronic pain. It can be used under the tongue (sublingual), in the cheek (buccal), by injection (intravenous), as a skin patch (transdermal), or as an implant. For opioid use disorder, it is typically started when withdrawal symptoms have begun and for the first two days of treatment under direct observation of a health-care provider.

Cannabinoids are compounds found in cannabis. The most notable cannabinoid is the phytocannabinoid tetrahydrocannabinol (THC) (Delta9-THC or Delta8-THC), the primary psychoactive compound in cannabis.

Codeine is an opiate and prodrug of morphine used to treat pain, coughing, and diarrhea and is commonly abused. It is found naturally in the sap of the opium poppy, Papaver somniferum. It is typically used to treat mild to moderate degrees of pain.

Cyclopentanophenanthrene (usually uncountable, plural cyclopentanophenanthrenes) (organic chemistry). The tetracyclic skeleton that, with a branched side chain, is common to all steroids.

Dopamine (DA, a contraction of 3, 4-dihydroxyphenethylamine) is a neurotransmitter that plays several important roles in the brain and body. It is an organic chemical of the catecholamine and phenethylamine families. Dopamine constitutes about 80% of the catecholamine content in the brain.

Hallucinogen is a psychoactive agent that often or ordinarily causes hallucinations, perceptual anomalies, and other substantial subjective changes in thought, emotion, and consciousness that are not typically experienced to such degrees with other drug classifications.

Hydrocodone, sold under the brand name Zohydro ER, among others, is an opioid used to treat severe pain of a prolonged duration, if other measures are not sufficient. It is also used as a cough suppressant in adults.

Methadone, sold under the brand names Dolophine and Methadose among others, is a synthetic opioid agonist used for opioid maintenance therapy in opioid dependence and for chronic pain management. Detoxification using methadone can be accomplished in less than a month, or it may be done gradually over as long as six months

Methamphetamine (contracted from N-methylamphetamine) is a potent central nervous system (CNS) stimulant that is mainly used as a recreational drug and less commonly as a second-line treatment for attention deficit hyperactivity disorder and obesity. Methamphetamine was discovered in 1893 and exists as two enantiomers: levo-methamphetamine and dextro-methamphetamine.

Misdemeanor (American English, spelled misdemeanour in British English) is any "lesser" criminal act in some common law legal systems.

Oxycodone, sold under the brand names Roxicodone and OxyContin (which is the extended release form) among others, is an opioid medication used for treatment of moderate to severe pain.

Paranoia is an instinct or thought process which is believed to be heavily influenced by anxiety or fear, often to the point of delusion and irrationality.[1] Paranoid thinking typically includes persecutory beliefs, or beliefs of conspiracy concerning a perceived threat towards oneself (i.e. the American colloquial phrase, "Everyone is out to get me"). Paranoia is distinct from phobias, which also involve irrational fear, but usually no blame.

Pharmacokinetics (from Ancient Greek pharmakon "drug" and kinetikos "moving, putting in motion"; see chemical kinetics), sometimes abbreviated as PK, is a branch of pharmacology dedicated to determine the fate of substances administered to a living organism. The substances of interest include any chemical xenobiotic such as: pharmaceutical drugs, pesticides, food additives, cosmetics, etc.

Phencyclidine or phenylcyclohexyl piperidine (PCP), also known as angel dust among other names, is a drug used for its mind-altering effects. PCP may cause hallucinations, distorted perceptions of sounds, and violent behavior. As a recreational drug, it is typically smoked, but may be taken by mouth, snorted, or injected.

Phenylephrine is a medication primarily used as a decongestant, to dilate the pupil, to increase blood pressure, and to relieve hemorrhoids. While marketed as a decongestant, taken by mouth at recommended doses it is of unclear benefit for hay fever. It can be taken by mouth, as a nasal spray, given by injection into a vein or muscle, or applied to the skin.

Pseudoephedrine (PSE) is a sympathomimetic drug of the phenethylamine and amphetamine chemical classes. It may be used as a nasal/sinus decongestant,

Psychoactive drug, psychopharmaceutical, or psychotropic drug is a chemical substance that changes nervous system function and results in alterations in perception, mood, consciousness, cognition, or behavior. These substances may be used medically; recreationally; to purposefully improve performance or alter one's consciousness; as entheogens for ritual, spiritual, or shamanic purposes; or for research.

Psychotherapy (also psychological therapy or talking therapy) is the use of psychological methods, particularly when based on regular personal interaction with adults, to help a person change behavior and overcome problems in desired ways. Psychotherapy aims to improve an individual's well-being and mental health, to resolve or mitigate troublesome behaviors, beliefs, compulsions, thoughts, or emotions, and to improve relationships and social skills.

Schizophrenia is a mental disorder characterized by continuous or relapsing episodes of psychosis.major symptoms include hallucinations (typically hearing voices), delusions, and disorganized thinking. Other symptoms include social withdrawal, decreased emotional expression, and apathy.

Sedative or tranquilliseris a substance that induces sedation by reducing irritabilityor excitement. They are CNS depressants and interact with brain activity causing its deceleration.

Tetrahydrocannabinol (THC) is the principal psychoactive constituent of cannabis and one of at least 113 total cannabinoids identified in the plant

BIBLIOGRAPHY

1991. *Drug abuse and drug abuse research.* Rockville, Md.: Dept. of Health and Human Services, Public Health Service, Alcohol, Drug Abuse, and Mental Health Administration, National Institute on Drug Abuse.

1994. *Epidemiologic trends in drug abuse.* Rockville, Md. (5600 Fishers Lane 20857): National Institutes of Health, Division of Epidemiology and Prevention Research, National Institute on Drug Abuse.

DrugAbuse.com. 2021. *Drug Abuse Treatment – Alcohol and Substance Abuse Programs.* [online] Available at: <https://drugabuse.com/?fbclid= IwAR2EEfolA9gk3AD_vW00wcVWNJv4UI_RFdFpmwYaBjS QcAcpYUpvTseryKo> [Accessed 16 June 2021].

Espejo, R., 2002. *Drug abuse*. San Diego, Calif.: Greenhaven Press.

Healthyplace.com. 2021. *What is Drug Abuse? Drug Abuse Information | HealthyPlace*. [online] Available at: <https://www.healthyplace.com/addictions/drug-addiction/what-is-drug-abuse-drug-abuse-information?fbclid=IwAR1ngV-8-kqZ2q5bd4NKglbujSJg1bIZCAevO97YQZANcWTl89Po2EXd HWw> [Accessed 16 June 2021].

Medicinenet.com. 2021. [online] Available at: <https://www.medicinenet.com/drug_abuse/article.htm?fbclid=IwAR0lvhcOpvyl0h4FuzOUfhrcuDpbpsyRrvpWGE5s-LfugRiW22Bbxynltk4> [Accessed 16 June 2021].

National Institute on Drug Abuse. 2021. *Drugabuse.gov | National Institute on Drug Abuse (NIDA)*. [online] Available at: <https://www.drugabuse.gov/?fbclid=IwAR2wnS0SLp8CvQqof4RD9aGPiAEMVEF82M3RB0Snhy M6fl8XgBnOROqSeoA> [Accessed 16 June 2021].

National Institute on Drug Abuse. 2021. *Understanding Drug Use and Addiction DrugFacts | National Institute on Drug Abuse*. [online] Available at: <https://www.drugabuse.gov/publications/drugfacts/understanding-drug-use-addiction?fbclid=IwAR0IEDzYO6KFYmBT0mbGKfFwDJIzzv5hj9w93myO8rQ kzqkpCjfpuLygEQw> [Accessed 16 June 2021].

WebMD. 2021. *Drug Addiction: Know the Warning Signs.* [online] Available at: <https://www.webmd.com/mental-health/addiction/drug-abuse-addiction?fbclid= IwAR2If4cYrFvcebOUGpaDvKFDFO5R0eaR3PcevNh2TkcZT 7Ch-Kj8MBqCmhY#1> [Accessed 16 June 2021].

WebMD. 2021. *Drug Addiction: Know the Warning Signs.* [online] Available at: <https://www.webmd.com/mental-health/addiction/drug-abuse-addiction?fbclid= IwAR25uhSq77In3NAvN0Gv7jtJsiXCvoOr-JMn_AFu770EVso9RLdZGj6DrvA#1> [Accessed 16 June 2021].

www.ingramcontent.com/pod-product-compliance
Lightning Source LLC
Chambersburg PA
CBHW030250030426
42336CB00009B/329